Yoga Stories for Kids

YOGA STORIES FOR KIDS:
A Path to Resilience and Growth

by Sharon Mond

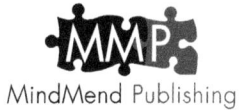
MindMend Publishing

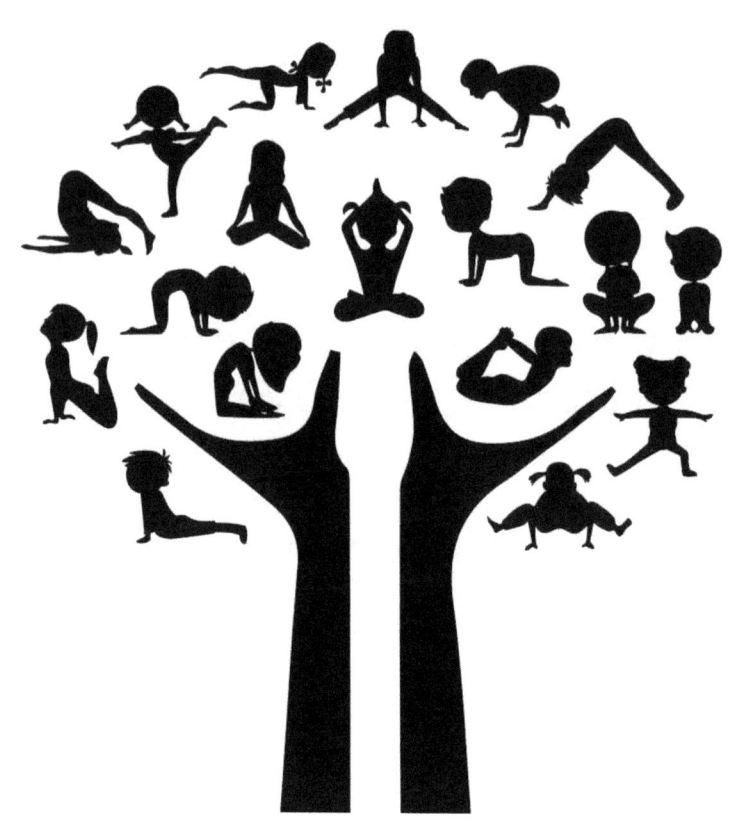

Published in 2018 by the MindMend Publishing Co., New York, NY
Copyright 2018 © by SharonMond.
All rights reserved.

For permissions to reproduce more than 150 words of this publication,
email to ORIPressEditor@gmail.com or write to MindMend Publishing Editor,
7515 187th Street, Fresh Meadows, NY 11366.

Printed in the United States of America on acid free paper.

Library of Congress Control Number: 2018967271

Cataloging Data:
Mond, Sharon. Yoga Stories for Kids: A Path to Resilience and Growth/ Sharon Mond.

1. Yoga. 2. Yoga for children. 3. Yoga – application in schools. 4. Yoga – therapeutic application. 5. Non-formal education. 6. Health & fitness – alternative therapies. 7. Body-mind therapies.

ISBN 978-1-942431-10-7 (soft cover)

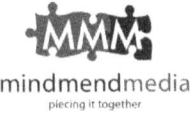

Book design, editing, and book cover –
byMindMendMedia, Inc. @ MindMendMedia.com

I would like to express my thanks and appreciation
to my husband, Michael Mond, whose
love,
support,
and encouragement
made this book possible.

Thank you to all the children
who have moved with me.

TABLE OF CONTENTS

Foreword……..xi

Preface……..xiii

Part I: **Yoga Poses**

Child Pose……..2

Mountain……..4

Chair Pose……..6

Tree……..8

Bird……..10

Butterfly……..12

Rabbit……..14

Cat/ Cow……..16

Downward Dog……..18

Lion……..20

Frog……..22

Snake……..24

Bear……..26

Eagle……..28

Turtle……..30

Horse……..32

Deer……..34

Snail……..36

Surox……..38

Owl……..40

Fish……..42

Elephant……..44

Warrior I……..46

Moon Beam……..48

Turkey……..50

Part II: **Primary Elementary Stories**

The Tree……..55

Lion's Secret……..57

The Roar……..59

Big Problem? Little Problem? A Lion Story……..63

The Great Commotion: A Lion Story……..67

The Lost Bear……..69

Part III: **Intermediate Elementary Stories**

Yoga Forest Story……..75

Jungle Story……..79

Thanksgiving……..83

Homer's Emergency……..85

Copying and Teasing……..91

The Mountain Climb……..95

The Seed Inside……..101

The Gate……..105

Moving On……..111

***Afterword*……..115**

FOREWORD

MindMend Publishing is excited to present to the world the *Yoga Stories* that are set to be a resource for parents, teachers, mentors, coaches, and ultimately – for children who (by definition of their age) are not well equipped to navigate through all the world's pitfalls. As Maurice Sendak, one of the most beloved children books' author and illustrator, once said, "Childhood is a very, very tricky business of surviving it. Because if…anything goes wrong, and usually something goes wrong, then you are compromised as a human being. You're going to trip over that for a good part of your life." Can this grim path into life be changed? What is the agent of change? Who would be in charge of such change? Usually, it is not the government, not the rules and regulations established by politicians, but the adults in a child's life that could make such a change, because the adults are the natural models for children's ways of being.

The concept of childhood has transformed tremendously since Oliver Twist's times, and today, it would be true to say that most parents are making sure that their children have a roof over their head, that they are healthy, and that they are achieving their educational goals. Still, many adults cannot recognize or deal with their children's worries, anxieties, and other (often insidious and silent) signs of that tricky business of childhood, especially when something has gone wrong. Traumatized children also tend to hide their unregulated emotions in their bodies, or they tend to dissociate – "because they can" – and no one in the world would know where they are hiding!

This small volume of *Yoga Stories* offers invaluable tools for an understanding of the non-verbal expressions of children's troubles, and for finding the correct language to first normalize, and then, stabilize and regulate children's feelings, emotions, and thoughts – which can often be overwhelming for them.

Yoga Stories can be used as an "emotion coach" that teaches children to appreciate their own bodies, the connection of their emotions to what they feel in their bodies, as well as self-regulation, a process very important in one's emotional development. Self-regulation leads to one's ability to expand their window of tolerance, to live creatively, to live in present moment, and not to be traumatized by various life events.

Reading *Yoga Stories* can be helpful for teachers and parents, as well as for children themselves, and on many levels. In addition to the yoga poses that help kids with self-regulation problems, the children are engaged in creative and imaginary work here. As in *The Wonderful Wizard of Oz*, the children also connect here with non-human creatures (and even with the parts of these creatures' characters, like the Lion's roar), all of which promote the very human values, teach kids many things about how to live emotionally healthy lives, and to form and maintain strong relationships with others.

Dr. Inna Rozentsvit,
on behalf of MindMend Publishing Co.

PREFACE

The stories in this collection were inspired by the children with whom I worked in a public school setting as a dance/movement therapist for students with behavioral, emotional, and developmental disorders. The *Yoga Stories* gave voice to the conflicts and issues that the students under my care were encountering, when they often did not have the words to express themselves. Feelings of loss, low self-esteem, identity, anger, bullying, anxiety, fear, friendship, overcoming obstacles, developing coping skills, and discovering hope – are all raised in the dilemmas faced by the characters in the stories.

The children I worked with were able to relate to the conflicts in the stories. They were able to understand that they are not alone in their experiences, and that there are positive ways to cope with them. Adding movement, Yoga, and imagery helped to take the children deeper into the process of healing, as it allowed them to access their mind and body, finding strength, peace, and resolution when facing difficulty.

The children loved the stories. They repeatedly asked me for more. They remembered the stories long after I presented them, and they often wanted to know more about the characters. I believe that the themes presented in these stories are universal, and they will appeal to elementary aged children in many settings.

The fifteen stories are divided into two categories: six stories are for the kindergarten through second grade age (primary elementary), and nine are for third through fifth grade (intermediate elementary).

The characters in the primary elementary stories are animals, each of which has a Yoga pose associated with it. Before sharing the stories, I taught the poses for each animal, and the children practiced them until they could do the movement when the name of the animal was called out. I presented the stories using puppets, and the children were able to do the poses while watching the puppets as they heard the story. Following the stories, we verbally processed the value, the social skills, and the feelings that were presented by the characters. The children were then given the opportunity to take turns using the puppets to retell the story – each in their own way. Finally, the children were offered paper and crayons, so that they could draw their own image of the story, and then share their drawing with the group. The stories in this category include: "Lion's Secret," "The Roar," "Big Problem? Little Problem? A Lion's Story," "The Great Commotion," "The Lost Bear," and "The Tree."

    The stories for the intermediate elementary grades contain animals, children, and adults as characters. As in the primary elementary stories, when an animal is a character here, it is also associated with a Yoga pose. This helped the story to become a bridge between the age groups as the children advanced through school. "Yoga Forest Story," "Jungle Story," and "Thanksgiving" are examples of stories that create that bridge. The other stories in this grouping use Yoga as the way to cope with problems and to self-regulate, and breathing and movements are written directly into the stories themselves. After presenting the stories to this age group, I followed up with questions about the values, social skills, and conflicts revealed in the story, offered mandalas or coloring pages that relate to visual imagery of the story, or suggested that children draw their own images connected to the story's themes. Stories of this grouping include: "Homer's Problem," "Copying and Teasing," "The Mountain Climb," "The Seed Inside," "The Gate," and "Moving On."

    It is my sincere hope and belief that these stories will resonate with children as they navigate the issues that are part of growing up, and that they will help children to cope with their adverse experiences and to communicate their feelings.

    A little about me: I am a Board Certified Dance/Movement Therapist (BC-DMT), a Licensed Professional Clinical Counselor (LCPC), a Nationally Certified Counselor (NCC), a Dance Educator (Maryland State Department of Education, Advanced Professional Certificate), a Yoga Instructor (RYT-200), and a painter.

Part I:
YOGA POSES

CHILD POSE
(Garbhasana)

Begin on hands and knees (Table pose). Sit back on the heels and lower the upper body to the legs. Arms can either rest along the floor in front of the body or can be tucked next to the legs with the hands resting near the feet. Place the forehead on the floor.

YOGA POSES

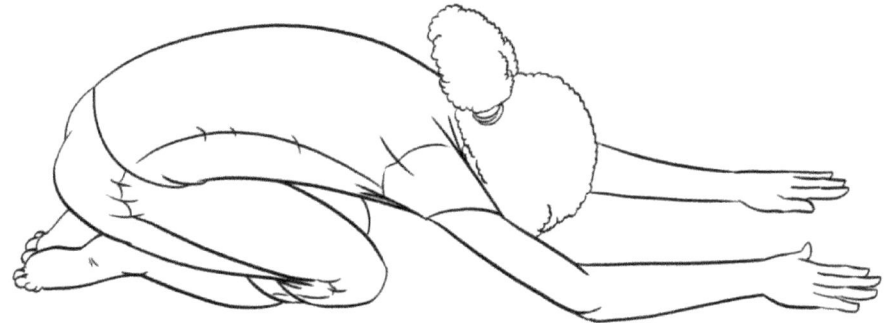

MOUNTAIN
(Tadasana)

Standing tall, feet parallel, ribs in, spine lengthened, chin parallel to the ground, breathing in the belly, arms down and slightly away from the body, palms forward.

YOGA POSES

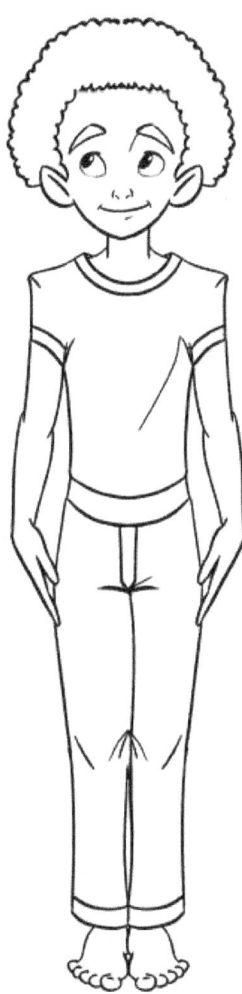

CHAIR POSE
(Utkatasana)

Begin in Mountain Pose. Inhale and raise the arms to shoulder height in front of the body, parallel to the floor, palms down. On the exhale, bend the knees, keeping the back long, with the belly in toward the spine to maintain length in the back. The upper body will lean forward in this pose. Relax the shoulders and breathe.

YOGA POSES

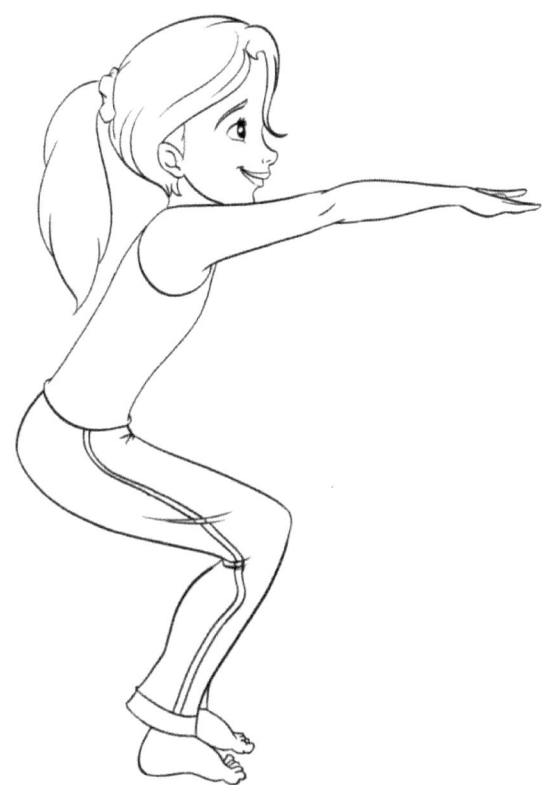

TREE
(Vriksasana)

This pose can be challenging for children. They can keep the toe of the raised foot on the floor to aid in balance. Standing on two feet, shift the weight onto the left foot. Place the heel of the right foot on the left ankle, or the right foot onto the left calf or thigh. Hands can be pressed together at the heart center. Once stability is achieved, the arms can be raised overhead.

YOGA POSES

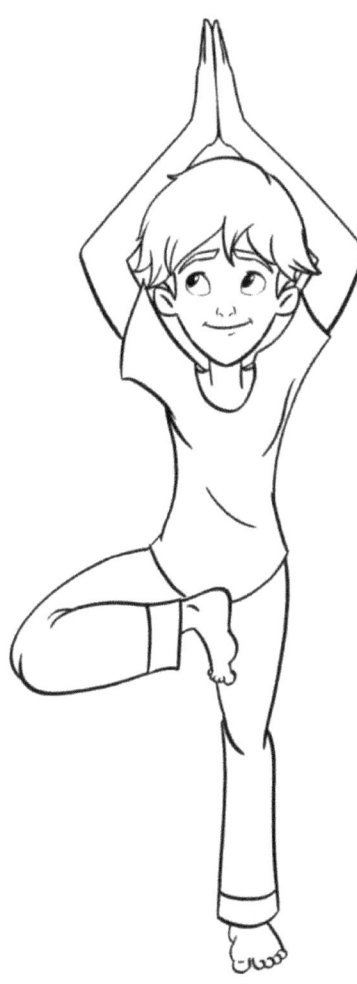

BIRD
(Warrior III pose, modified Virabhadrasana)

Standing on one leg, bend the torso forward while extending the other leg directly behind you, balancing on the standing leg. Open the arms to the sides. This is a challenging pose. For young children, the pose can be modified by standing on both legs with the arms open to the side at shoulder height.

YOGA POSES

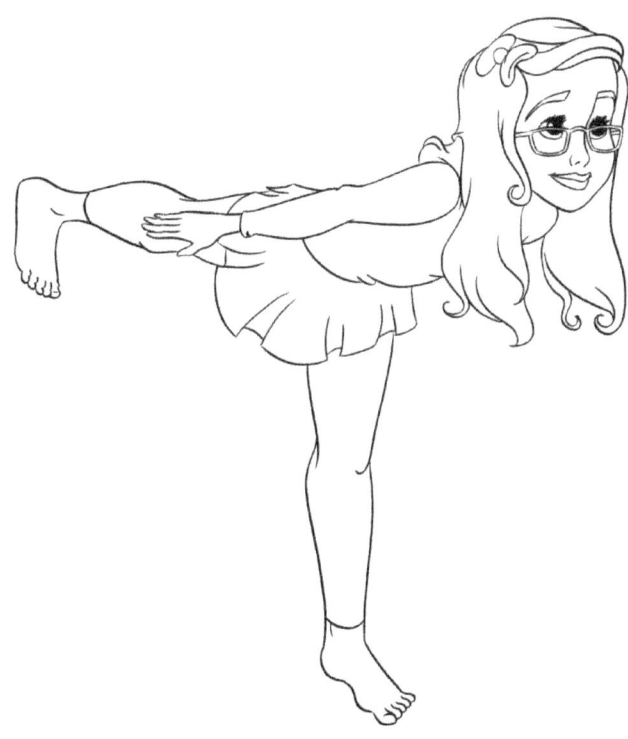

BUTTERFLY
(Baddha Konasana)

Sitting on the floor, bring the soles of the feet together while maintaining a long back. Shoulders should be aligned over the pelvis. Bend the arms, with elbows out to the side of the body, and place the fingertips on the shoulders. The children can raise and lower their elbows on the inhale and exhale like a butterfly moves its wings.

YOGA POSES

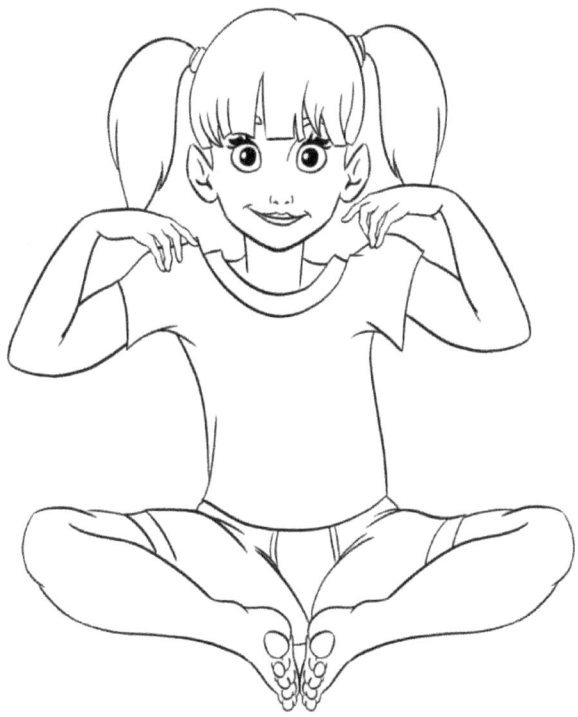

RABBIT
(Shashangasana)

Begin kneeling in Child Pose: upper body resting on the upper legs, forehead to the floor, arms close to the legs behind the body.

Tuck the top of the head close to the knees and clasp the hands together behind the back.

Breathe in and lift up onto the knees, keeping the top of the head in contact with the floor, while lifting the clasped hands above the back.

Breathe out to return to child's pose.

YOGA POSES

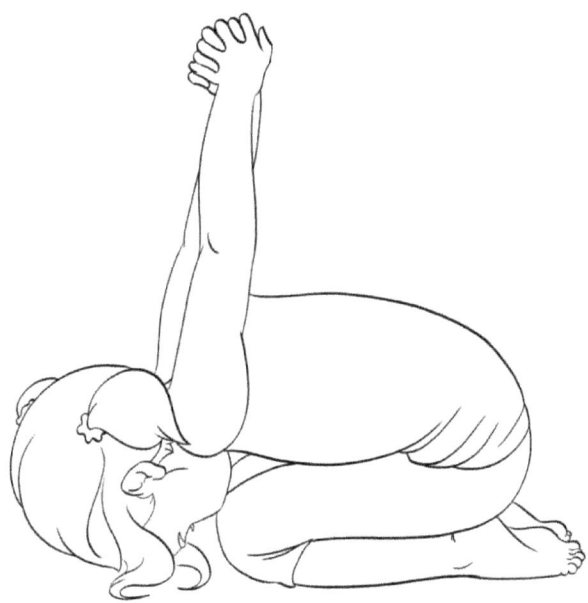

CAT & COW
(Marjariasana & Bitilasana)

Starting on hands and knees, breathe in and lift the head toward the sky while tilting the pelvis down so the belly dips toward the floor (cow).

Breathe out and arch the back to the sky while the head dips toward the floor (cat).

YOGA POSES

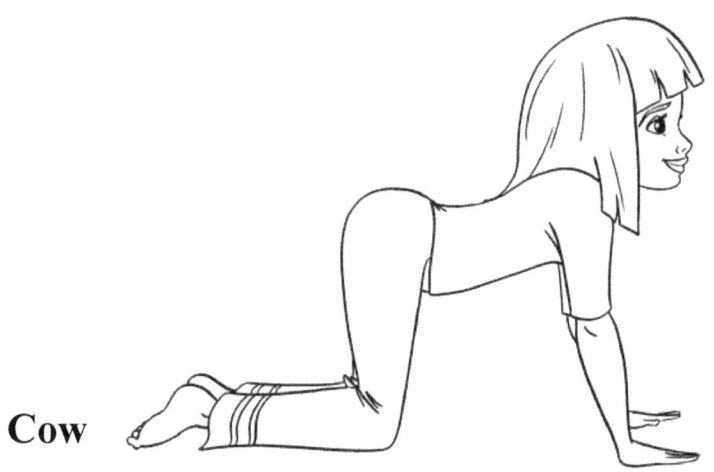

Cow

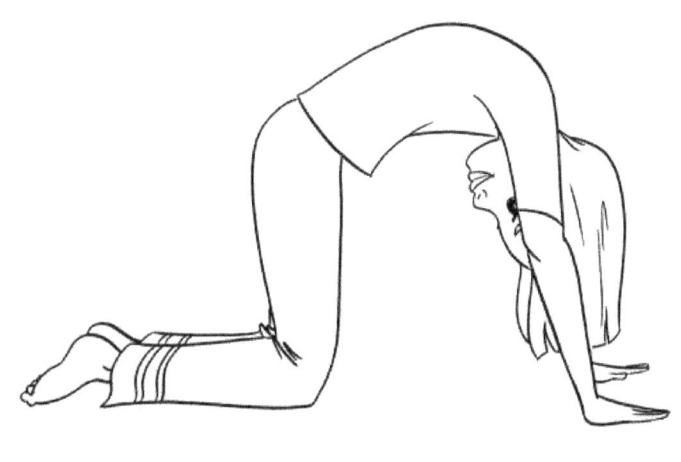

Cat

DOWNWARD DOG
(Adho Mukha Svanasana)

Begin in hands and knees position on the floor (Table). Move both hands slightly forward, and then curl the toes under the feet. With an inhale, press into the toes to lift the knees off the floor, lengthening the legs behind you. On the exhale press back toward the heels of the foot, keeping all five fingers, finger pads, and the outer edge of the hands pressing into the floor, creating an upside-down "V" posture.

YOGA POSES

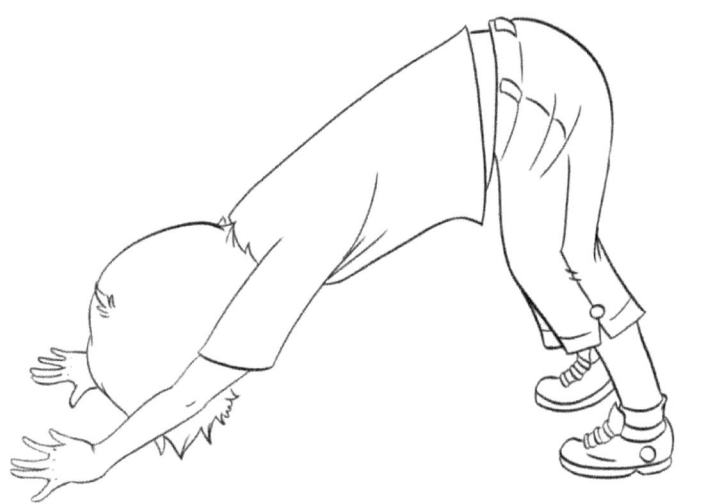

LION

Sit in traditional Hero Pose (Virasana) kneeling, sitting on heels, back is upright, hands rest on thighs.
Breathe in.
As you exhale, bend forward so that the chest folds towards the knees, keeping the elbows in toward the chest, while making a roaring sound.

YOGA POSES

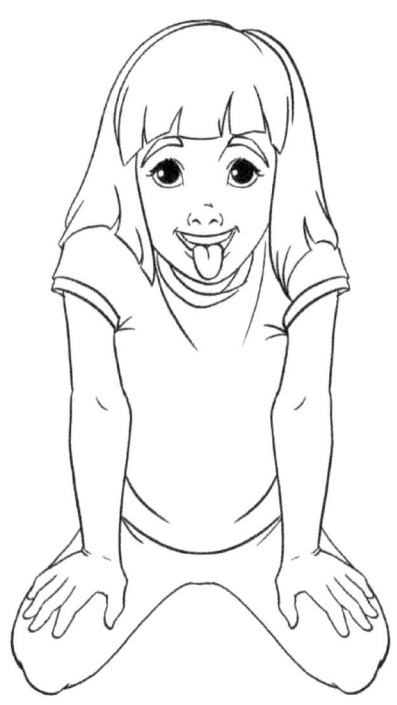

FROG
(Squat, Malasana)

Begin in a wide legged standing pose, with hands touching in front of the chest in prayer position. Breathe in and bend the knees into a squat while exhaling. Keep the back upright. Try to widen the legs enough, so that the heels remain on the floor. The elbows can touch the inner thigh to help support the pose.

YOGA POSES

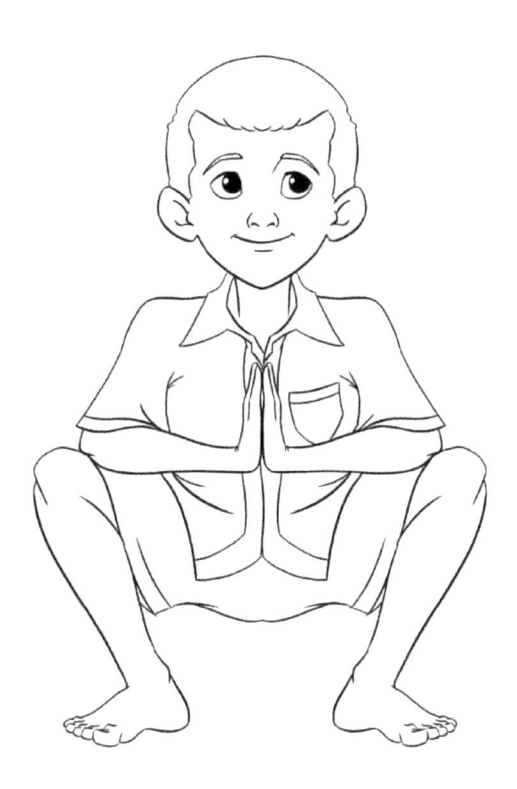

SNAKE
(Cobra, Bhujangasana)

Lying prone on the abdomen, place the hands under the shoulders, with the elbows close to the sides of the body.
Breathe in and press the hands into the floor while lifting the upper body off the floor. Hips should remain on the floor. Lengthen through the back to avoid compression on the lower back. As you lower your upper body to the floor, breathe out and make a hissing sound.

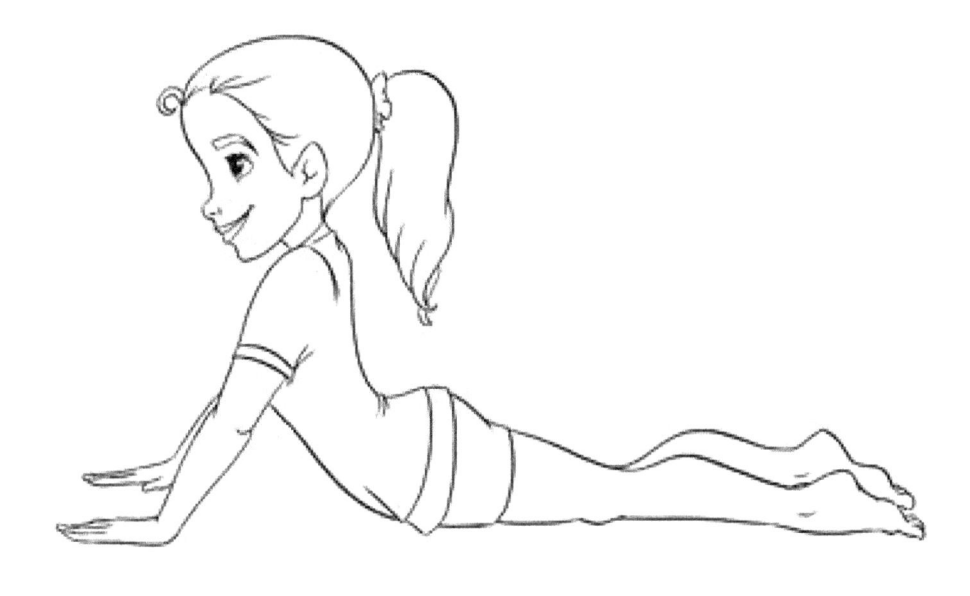

YOGA POSES

BEAR
(Star Pose, Utthita Tadasana, to Goddess Pose, Deviasana)

Begin by standing with wide legs, toes pointed away from the body, arms overhead, opened from the center.
Breathe in, and then as you exhale bend the knees and the elbows into Goddess pose, while growling.

YOGA POSES

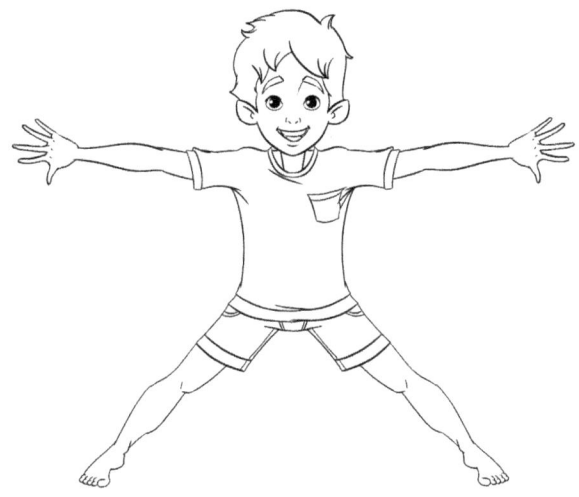

Star

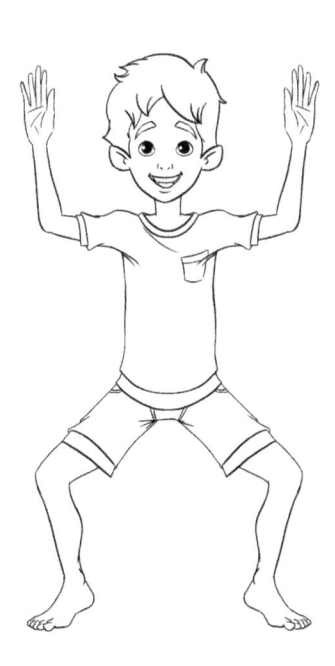

Goddess

EAGLE
(Garudasana)

This is a challenging pose for children. It is best to keep the toe of the raised foot onto the ground for support. Arms can be simplified by grasping them together in front of the body instead of twisting them in opposition to the legs as in the full expression of the pose.

Starting in standing pose (Tadasana), shift onto the left leg, bend the knee, and cross the right leg over the left (as mentioned above, for children, keep the toe of the right leg on the floor).

Squeeze the legs together.

The arms can be brought together, hands clasped, forearms pressing together in front of the body, or left arm crosses over the right, twinging the hands so that the palms are clasped together. Squeeze the arms.

Breathe in and out, and then breathe out to come out of the pose and repeat on the other side.

YOGA POSES

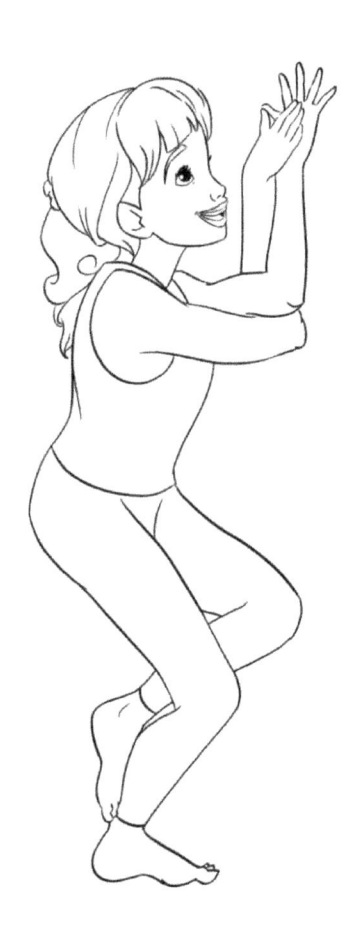

TURTLE

Seated in Bound Angle Butterfly Pose (Baddha Konasana), slip the arms under the knees.
Breathe in and then lean forward on the exhale, rounding the back over the legs while allowing the arms to extend under the legs.

YOGA POSES

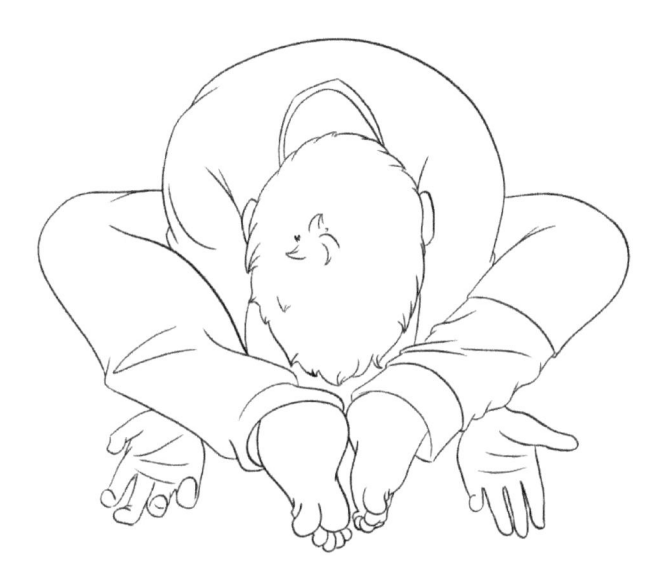

HORSE

This is a galloping movement. Make a "neigh" sound while moving.

YOGA POSES

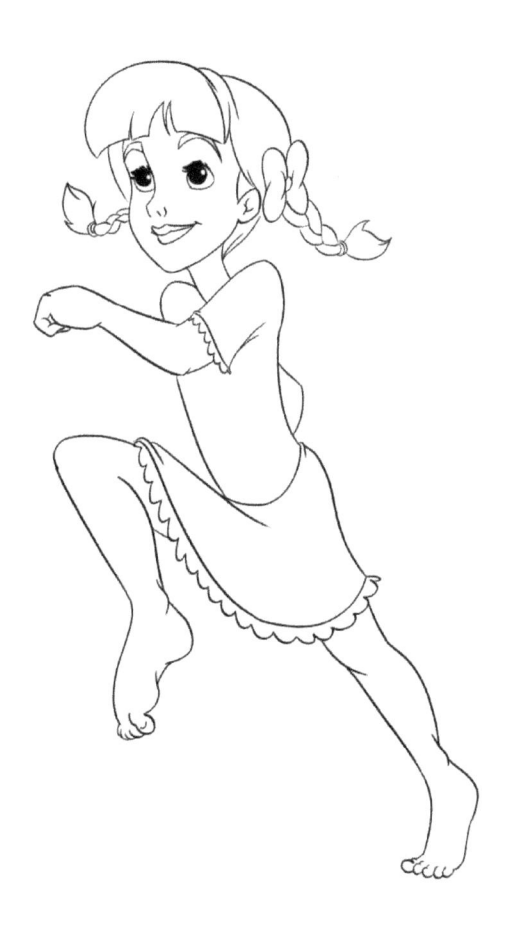

DEER

This is a galloping movement like by horse, but the hands are open, touching the top of the head like antlers.

YOGA POSES

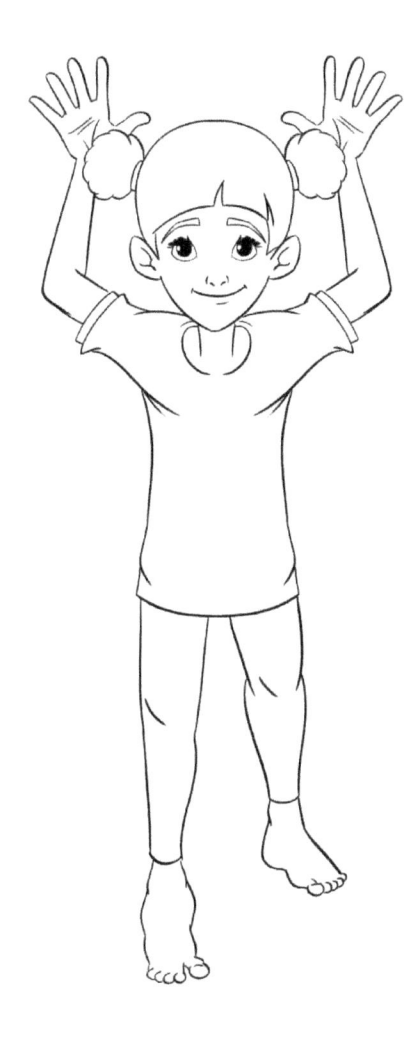

SNAIL
(modified Table Pose Marjariasana)

Starting on hands and knees (Table), lower the elbows to the floor and lower the forehead to the floor. Extend the arms forward. Breathe.

YOGA POSES

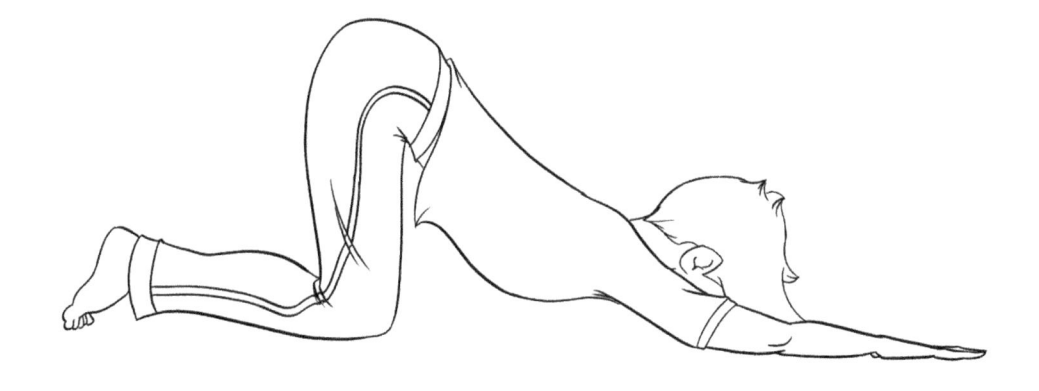

SUROX

My image of this imaginary creature is of an elevated Star Pose (Utthita Tadasana).

Standing with legs wide, arms wide above the head, rise on tiptoes then curl the hands forward while bending the knees and rounding the upper body forward, creating a rounded claw-like upper body shape.

YOGA POSES

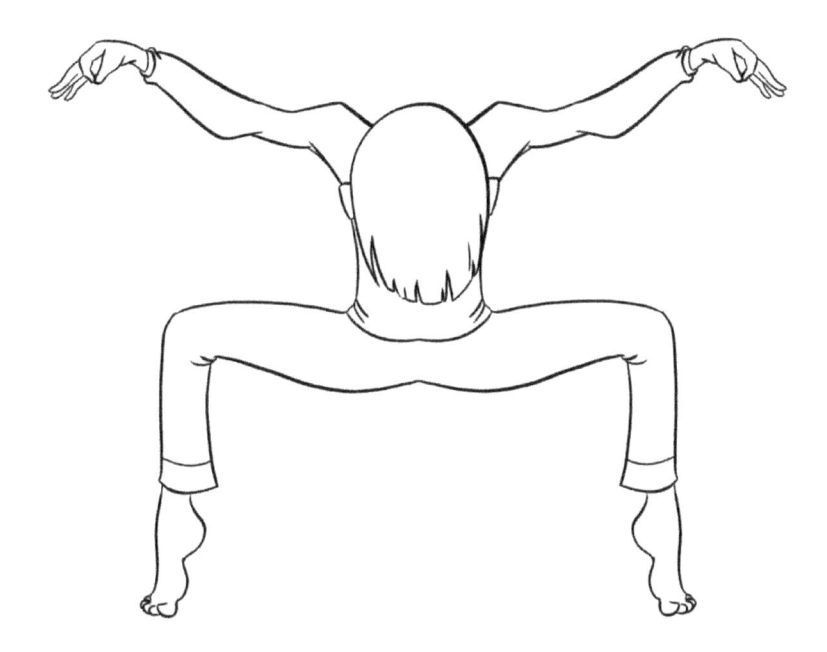

OWL
(Hero Pose, Virasana)

Begin by sitting on knees and lower legs, feet tucked in under the hips, and hands resting on top of the thighs. Slowly turn the head right and left as if nodding "no".

YOGA POSES

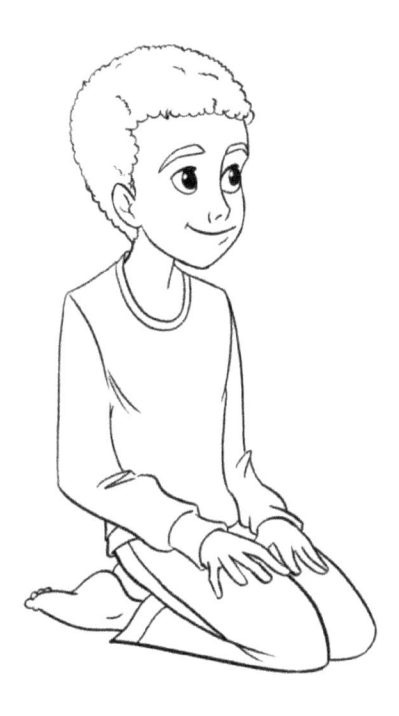

FISH
(Adaptation of the Boat Pose, Navasana)

Begin by lying prone on the floor, with the arms extended in front of the body, hands clasped together.

On an inhale, lift the arms and legs away from the floor. Arms can remain clasped together or parallel to each other.

I suggested to the children that they then wiggle their body while in this pose. On the exhale, lower the arms and legs back to the floor.

YOGA POSES

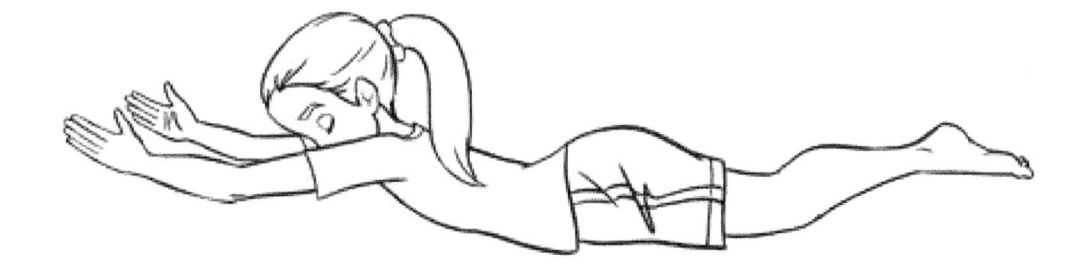

ELEPHANT

Begin by standing in a wide legged stance, arms to the side of the body.
To enter the pose, bend forward from the waist, clasping the hands together, and swing the arms from side to side, then front to back as if they were an elephant moving its trunk.

YOGA POSES

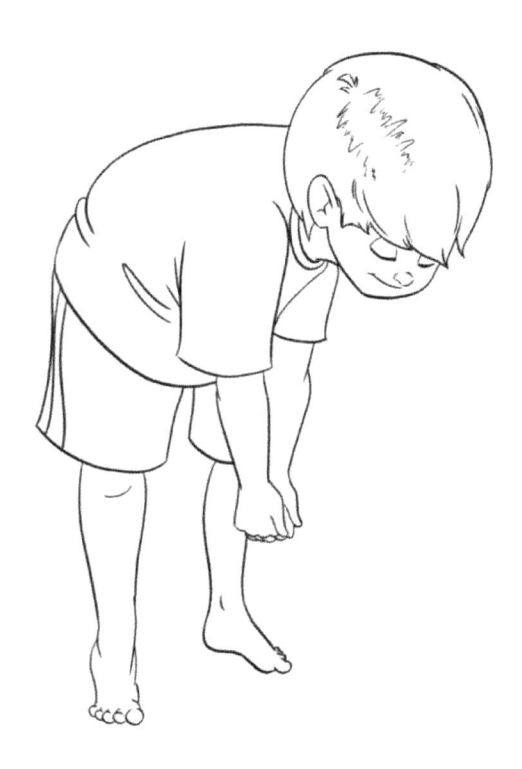

WARRIOR I
(Virabhadrasana I)

Starting in a standing Mountain Pose, step the right foot forward into a lunge, the back leg can rotate to allow the left foot to remain fully on the floor.
Bend the right knee so that the knee is directly above the right foot.
Extend the arms above the head. Breathe.
Step the feet together and repeat on the other side.

YOGA POSES

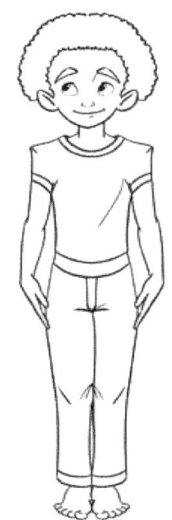

Mountain

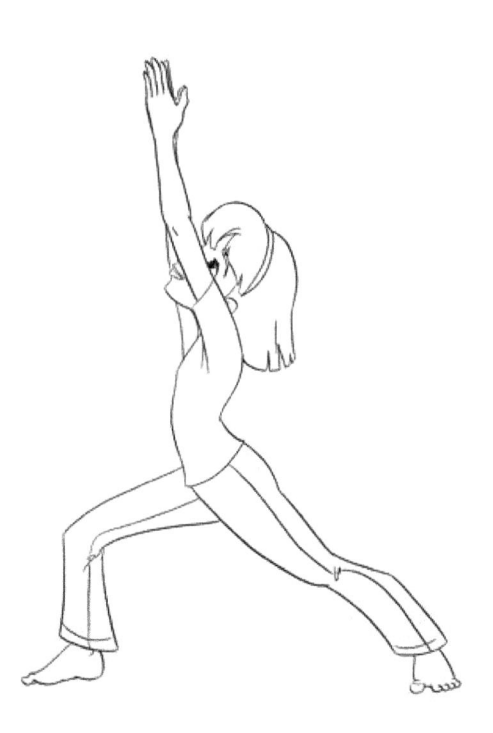

Warrior I

MOON BEAM
(Goddess, Deviasana, or Half Moon, Ardha Chandrasana)

To enter into Half Moon, begin in Mountain Pose.
Raise the arms and clasp them overhead. Lift the spine on an inhale, and bend the upper body to the right, exhale. Inhale to return to center and repeat on the other side.

YOGA POSES

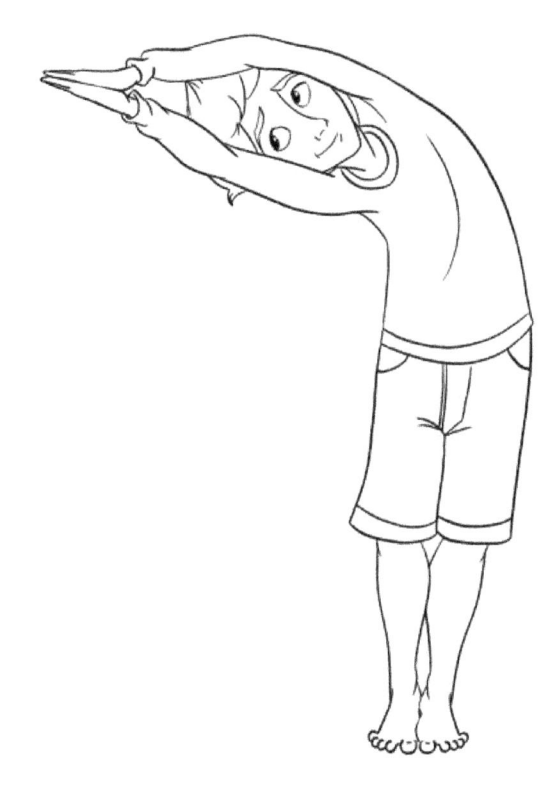

TURKEY
(Modified Squat, Malasana)

Start in a wide legged standing position, hands at heart center. Lower to squat and then move the squat side to side, forward and back.

YOGA POSES

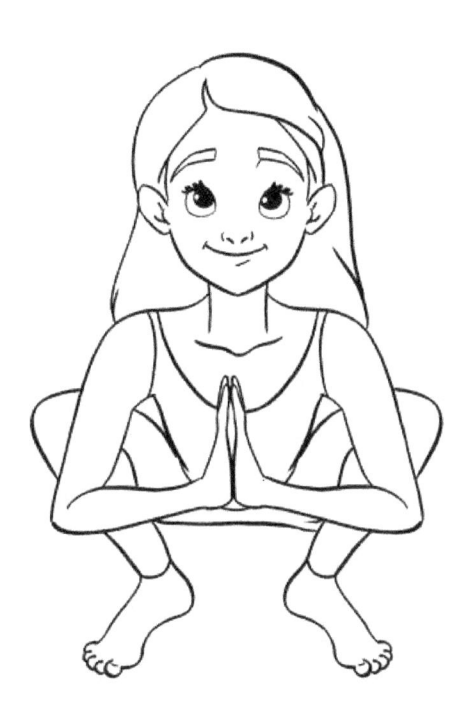

Part II:
PRIMARY ELEMENTARY STORIES
(Pre-Kindergarten - Second Grade)

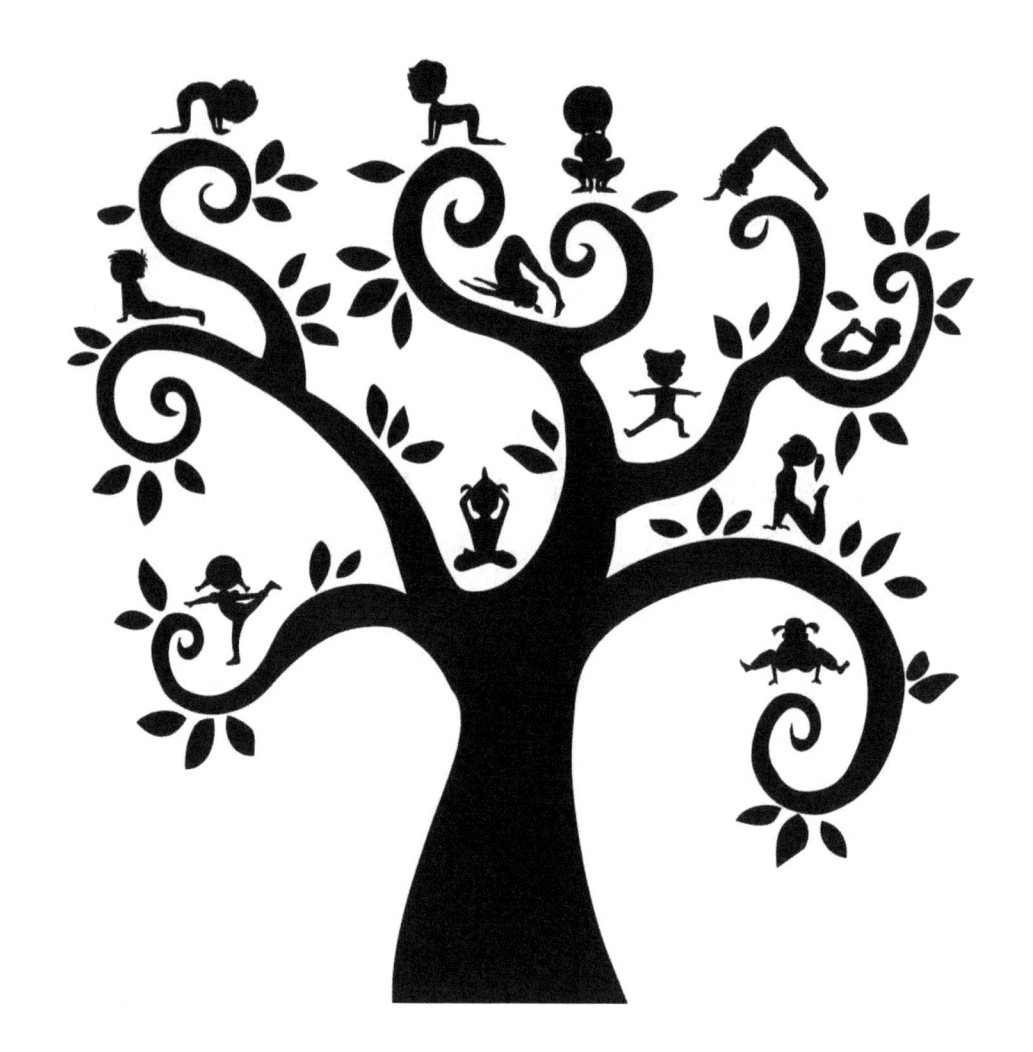

THE TREE

Once upon a time there was a little seed. The rain came and the sun came and the little seed grew and grew. Slowly, slowly, it grew until it became a tall tree, with many branches. Leaves grew on the branches and soon there were flowers. The flowers grew into cherries and the tree was happy.

One day a bird came by. It flew around and around the tree and then landed on its branches. The tree offered its fruit and the bird and tree were happy. The next day, a butterfly came to the tree. It fluttered its wings in and out and then landed on a branch of the tree. The tree offered its fruit and the butterfly and the tree were happy.

The next day, a bunny hopped by. It looked up the tree and down the tree. It hopped around the tree and stopped to sniff it. The tree dropped a cherry on the ground and the bunny began to nibble it. The bunny and the tree were happy.

Sometime later, the tree heard a sweet sound. "Meow, Meow." It was a cat. The cat arched its back and rubbed against the tree. It started to scratch and then climb the tree, and it climbed to the very top. On its way the cat picked up a cherry in its mouth and then stopped to eat it. The cat loved the cherry and started to purr. The cat and the tree were happy. Not long after that a dog came by. "Ruff, Ruff," it said, because it smelled the cat in the tree. The dog stretched and then circled around the tree. The tree let some cherries fall, and the dog ate them. The dog and the tree were happy.

But then the winds came. The winds grew stronger and stronger. The bird and the butterfly flew away, the bunny hopped away, and the cat and the dog ran away. The wind was so strong that the cherries fell down and were swept away. When the winds stopped the tree was very sad. It was afraid that its animal friends would not want to come anymore because there were no more cherries to eat. But guess what happened!

The bird flew back and said, "Can I still rest on your arms?"
The butterfly came by and said, "Can I still relax on your branches?"
The bunny came by and said, "Can I still curl up at your feet?"
The cat came by and said, "Can I still climb up to the top and curl up to sleep?"
The dog came by and said, "Can I still run and stretch and sit here below?"
The tree said, "Oh, Yes!"
And the bird, the butterfly, the bunny, the cat, the dog, and the tree were very happy.

DISCUSSION QUESTIONS FOR "THE TREE"

1. The tree, the bird, the butterfly, the bunny, the cat and the dog were very happy together. What made the animals go away? (The wind.)
2. How did the tree feel when the animals went away? (Very sad.)
3. Did the tree think the animals would come back? (No.) Why? (Because it didn't have any more cherries to give them.)
4. Did the animals come back? (Yes.) How did the tree feel? (Happy.)
5. What did the tree learn? (The tree learned that it did not have to give his friends something to like it, they liked the tree just for who it was.)

LION'S SECRET

There was a Lion who lived in the woods on the other side of the great meadow. He looked strong and fierce, and his roar was really loud. But Lion had a secret. He was scared. Really scared. Scared all the time. He roared really loud, so that others wouldn't know how scared he really was. He was afraid to ask for help when he was scared because he thought others would laugh at him. You see, everyone thinks Lions are brave all the time. But Lion did not feel that way.

Lion was scared of loud noises (ones he didn't make himself), of animals he had not met before, and he was scared of the dark. So, when he heard a loud noise or met a new creature, he roared really loud; and when it turned dark, he roared really loud; and then he went to find a place to hide. He didn't want anyone to know his secret. He felt embarrassed.

Bird was Lion's friend, but he didn't really like that Lion roared so loud each day. He decided that he would just have to say something.

"Lion, I noticed that yesterday, when a new friend, Dog, came by, you roared really loud. Why did you do that?"

Lion was afraid to say.

"And Lion," Bird said, "in the rainstorm the other day, you roared really loud. Why?"

Lion stayed quiet.

"And I hear you at night when I am trying to go to sleep. Can you please cut it out?" asked Bird.

Lion sighed.

"I'm trying, but I'm, I'm..."

"What is it?" asked Bird.

"I'm scared!" said Lion.

"Oh," Bird said. "I get it. Now I understand. Well, here's what we can do. Name something you like, and then think about it when you get scared. It will help you feel better."

"OK. Well, I like to see the sun rise. I will try to think about that when I feel scared next time," said Lion.

So, the next time Lion heard a noise, met a new creature, or was in the dark, he thought about the sun rise and – you know what – it helped! Just a little, at first, and then, the more he did it, the more it helped.

Maybe you can try it to the next time you feel scared.

DISCUSSION QUESTIONS FOR "LION'S SECRET"

1. Lion looked really strong and scary. How did Lion really feel? (Scared).
2. Why did Lion feel that way? (Lion was afraid that others would laugh at him.)
3. Did Lion try to hide his feelings? (Yes). How did Lion hide them? (He roared really loud.)
4. What did lion's friend, Bird do to help Lion? (He talked to him about his loud roar. He listened to Lion. He helped him find a way to feel better when he was scared.)
5. What did Bird tell Lion to do when he felt scared? (Think about something you like when you are scared.)
6. Did that idea help Lion? (Yes. The more he did it, the more it helped.)
7. Can we practice that idea too? (Give the children a chance to name something they like, so that they can think about it when they are scared. They can write it down or they can draw a picture of it, to keep it with them all the time.)

THE ROAR

Lion had a problem. He just knew it was a big problem, and he was scared. He didn't know what to do. He wanted to run, and Roar, but he couldn't. That was the problem. He had lost his Roar and he couldn't find it!

He looked under rocks, but his Roar wasn't there. He looked above at the trees, but his Roar wasn't there. He went to the pond, but his Roar wasn't there. He sat down and felt like crying.

Bird came by and saw that Lion was upset.

"What's the matter Lion," said Bird. "You look really upset."

"I lost my Roar," cried Lion. "I can't find it and I want it back. It is a really big problem! Without my Roar I can't warn my family and friends of danger, or show my strength. I need my Roar!"

"That is a really big problem," said Bird. "But you won't find it by looking under the rocks, or above at the trees, or even at the pond. That Roar is inside of you. Maybe we need to go to the Doctor!?"

Lion felt like crying. Without his Roar he couldn't feel his strength. "I guess you're right, Bird," said Lion. "Will you go with me? I think I need help."

"Sure, I'll go with you," said Bird. And off they went to see the Doctor.

When they arrived at the Doctor's office, it was a little busy, so they had to wait for a while. "I'm scared," said Lion to Bird.

"I'm here with you Lion," said Bird. "We will do this together."

Soon it was time to see the Doctor. "What seems to be the problem, Lion?" he asked. "How can I help you?"

"Doctor, I have lost my Roar. I can't find it anywhere," said Lion.

"Hum," said the Doctor, rubbing his chin. "I hear that you can talk, and I see that you can breathe well. Let me look in your throat."

The Doctor took out his little flashlight and looked way down into Lion's throat.

"Well it does look red," the Doctor said. "Have you been roaring a lot recently?"

"Yes, I guess I have," said Lion. "There have been so many things that have made me angry! Frog tried to copy my Roar, and that made me angry. Snake tried to take my snack, and that made me angry. Bear got in my favorite cave, and that made me angry. I just had to Roar!"

"Well, that's why you lost your Roar," said the Doctor. "You were using it so much it just got used up! You need to give your Roar a rest. You need to talk to Frog and Snake and Bear and solve problems with them, not just roar at them!"

"I guess you are right, Doctor," said Lion. "I will talk to them and try to solve the problems."

Lion went home, and thought about what the Doctor said. He decided he would talk to his friends the very next day.

Lion went to see Frog. He said, "I'm sorry I roared at you Frog. I was upset because you tried to copy my Roar, and this is my very special sound. I don't like it when someone tries to copy my Roar."

"I didn't know that," said Frog. "Now that I know, I won't do it again. Can we still be friends?"

"Yes," said Lion. And Lion and Frog were both happy.

"That was not as big of a problem as I thought," said Lion. "I feel happy. I will try to find Snake next."

Lion went to look for Snake and found him under a tree.

"Snake, I'm sorry I roared at you. I was angry because you took my snack. I was really hungry, and I get grumpy when I am hungry. Please don't take my snack again," said Lion.

"I'm sorry, Lion. I didn't mean to upset you. I was also really hungry and I saw your snack sitting there, and I just grabbed it. I guess, I could have found my own snack, but I didn't think about it at the time. I won't take your snack again," said Snake.

"Ok, thanks for telling me what you were feeling. I forgive you," said Lion.

"Friends?" asked Snake.

"Friends," replied Lion.

Lion was really happy. "Another problem solved," he thought. "Now I will find Bear."

Lion went into the woods near the caves to look for Bear. It took a while, but Lion found him sitting just inside a cave near the river.

"I'm sorry I roared at you, Bear," Lion said. "You made me really angry when you went into my cave to take your nap. That is my special place, and I don't like it when others are in there."

"I'm sorry too," said Bear. "I was just so sleepy that I went into the first cave I found. I didn't think about it being your special place. I can understand how you want your own space. I will do my best not to go into your space again."

"Thanks for understanding, Bear. I will do my best not to roar right away when I get upset. I will try to figure out how to solve the problem. It looks like I can solve problems with others instead of just getting angry. I know I will have to practice solving problems with others, but I think I can do it."

"That sounds great, Lion. I will do it too. Friends?" asked Bear.

"Friends," said Lion.

The next day Lion went back to the Doctor.

"Doctor, thank you so much for helping me! I have my Roar back, and not only that – I have solved my problems with Frog, Snake, and Bear! The problems were not as big as I thought!"

"I am happy for you, Lion," said the Doctor. "It is always good to really look at the problem, and then decide how you react to it. Most of the time, a problem is not as big as you think it is, and you can solve it when you stay calm. I hope you have learned your lesson."

"I have," said Lion. "I know I will need to practice it, but I will do better next time."

DISCUSSION QUESTIONS FOR "THE ROAR"

1. What was Lion's problem? (He lost his Roar.)
2. How did he feel? (Really upset.)
3. How did Bird help him? (Bird took him to the Doctor.)
4. Why did Lion lose his Roar? (He was angry a lot, and he used his Roar too much!)
5. What did Lion learn that he could do instead of roaring when he was angry? (He could talk to the creatures he was upset with, explain why he was upset, and work with them to solve his problems.)
6. What else did he learn? (Some problems are small, and some problems are big. You can solve small problems by talking them out and staying calm. It is good to take a breath and really look at the problem before reacting.)

PART II: PRIMARY ELEMENTARY STORIES

BIG PROBLEM? LITTLE PROBLEM?
A LION STORY

"I have a problem," said Lion to his friend Bird. "And, I don't know if it is a big problem or a little problem."

"Well, maybe I can help you," said Bird. "What is the problem?"

"Every day I go down to the pond to drink some water, and every day at the same time I get there, Bear is there too to drink some water."

"So, what is the problem with that?" asks Bird.

"Bear goes to my favorite spot to drink his water!" replies Lion. "I get really annoyed! I don't know what to do. Is this a big problem or a small problem?" asks Lion.

"Hum…, let me think," says Bird. "Bear is in the space you like to go to when you drink water. Hum… I think that is a small problem."

"Why?" asks Lion. "It feels like a big problem to me. I get really annoyed. I feel like roaring!"

"It is a small problem because you can solve it easily. You can simply ask Bear if he can move over a bit, so that you can both drink," says Bird.

"Well, what if he won't move over?" asks Lion.

"Then you can ask him to take turns with you," replies Bird. "One day you could drink first, and the next day Bear could drink first. That way it is fair to you both."

"Wow, you have two solutions to the same problem! I will talk to Bear tomorrow when I go down to the pond. Thank you for helping me Bird. I see now that this is a small problem. I don't have to get so angry that I want to roar," said Lion.

The next day Lion went down to the pond, and he saw Bear walking toward the water at the same time.

"Bear," said Lion, "I have a little problem that I want to talk to you about."

"What is it Lion?" said Bear.

"You and I come to the same spot every morning to drink from the pond. This is my favorite spot and there is not enough room for us to drink there at the same time. Do you think you could move over a little bit so that we could both drink, but I could still drink in my favorite place?" asked Lion.

Bear thought for a moment and said, "I don't mind moving over. I didn't even know that this was your favorite spot or that it bothered you. Thanks for telling me, Lion."

Lion felt really happy that he was able to talk to Bear about his problem and solve it without getting angry. It really was a little problem, but it was still important to him.

"Thank you, Bear. I am happy that we could solve the problem together," said Lion.

"Me too," said Bear.

They both smiled and drank.

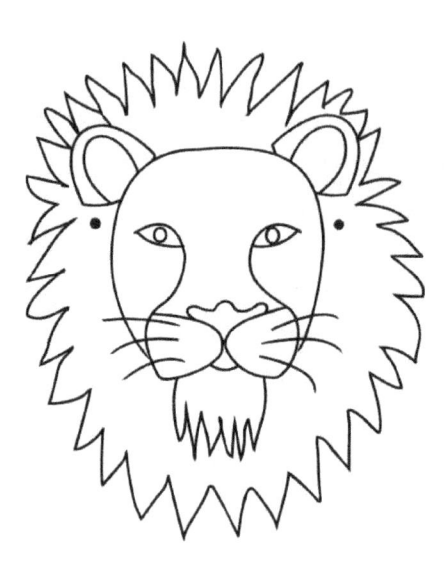

PART II: PRIMARY ELEMENTARY STORIES

DISCUSSION QUESTIONS FOR "BIG PROBLEM? LITTLE PROBLEM? A LION STORY"

1. What was Lion's problem in this story? (Bear wants to drink water in Lion's spot.)
2. How did Bird help Lion? (Bird helped Lion see that this was not a big problem, and that there were two ways he could solve the problem.)
3. Was Lion able to solve the problem with Bear? (Yes!)
4. How did Lion feel when he and Bear solved the problem? (Happy.)
5. Do you think there could be more than one way to solve a problem? (Yes, for sure.)
6. This can be an opportunity to talk to the children about problems they have in the classroom and work with them on one or two ways to solve the problem.

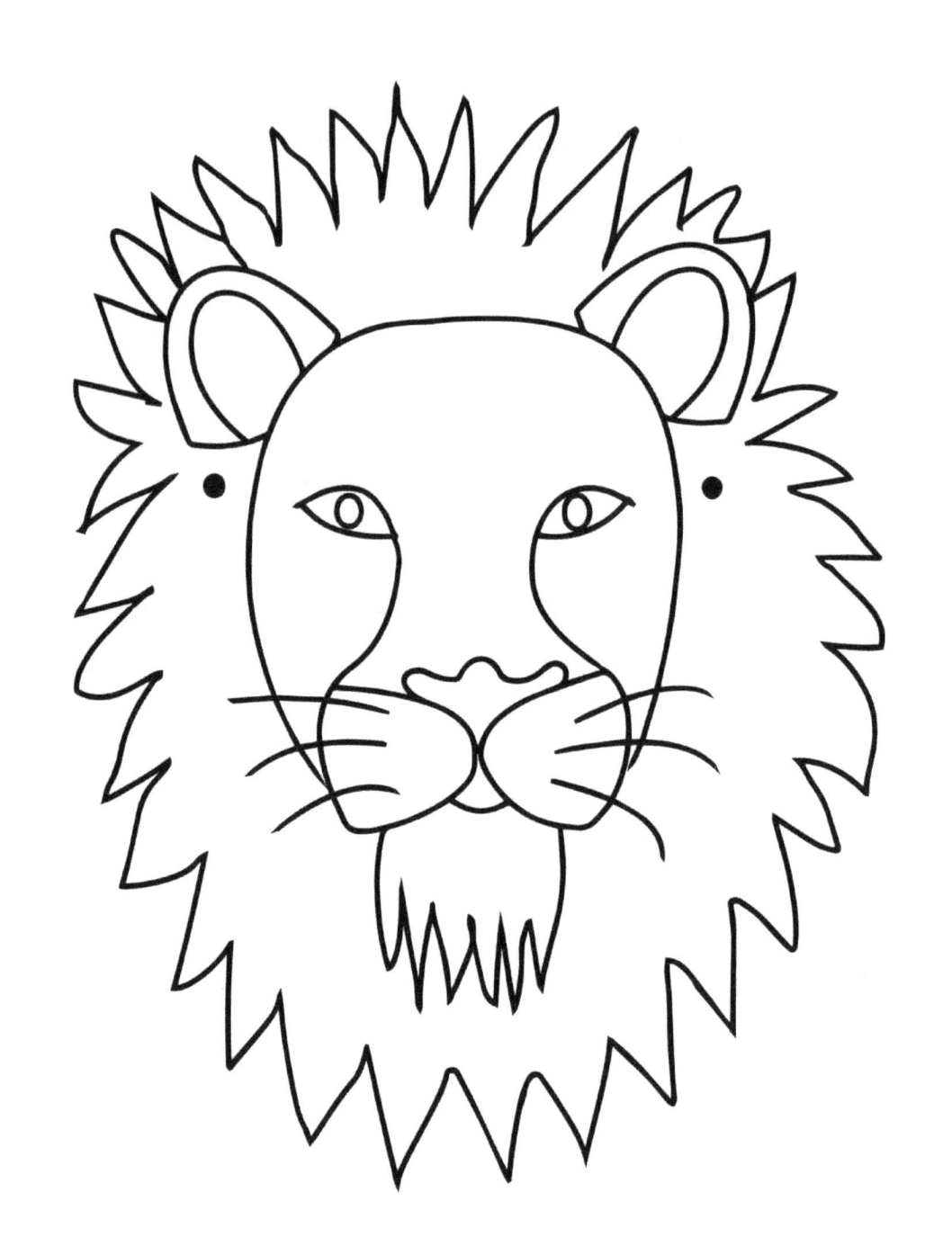

PART II: PRIMARY ELEMENTARY STORIES

THE GREAT COMMOTION: A LION STORY

One day Lion was walking in the woods when he heard a great commotion.
What is a "commotion?" It is a lot of noise.
"Squawk, Squawk, Caw, Caw, Hiss, Hiss!"
It sounded just terrible!
Lion ran toward the noise. He couldn't believe what he saw when he got there.
Bird was circling around Snake and was trying to bite him! Snake was hissing and trying to get away from Bird.
Bird was saying, "I don't like you Snake. I'm going to get you!"
Lion called out, "Bird, Snake, what is going on? Stop it right now!"
Bird said, "I don't like Snake. He is different. He can't fly. He slithers on the ground. I don't like that!"
Snake said, "Yeah, well I don't like you either."
They began to snarl, snap, hiss, and glare at each other, and then they tried to fight again.
"Stop that," said Lion. "Both of you!"
Just then, Frog hopped by and said, "I heard the noise. What's going on?"
Bear joined them and said, "I was sleeping in my cave and I heard the racket. You guys woke me up. What's happening?"
Bunny came by next and said, "You all scared me! Why are you so loud?"
Lion said, "Bird and Snake are fighting, and they won't stop! Help me solve this problem."
What do YOU think they should do?
Lion and Bear held onto Bird, and Bunny and Frog held onto Snake.
"Now," said Lion, "Bird and Snake, you will each get a chance to talk."

Bird answered, "I don't like Snake. He is different than me."

Snake replied, "I feel bad that he doesn't like me. I was born this way. I can't help the way I am."

"You both need to be kind to each other," said Lion. "You don't have to like everyone, but you need to be kind and get along. Not everyone will be the same as you."

"I will try," said Bird. "I really don't like to fight."

"I can be kind," said Snake. "I don't want to fight either."

And from that day on, Bird and Snake did not fight. They were not always the best of friends, but they were kind and respectful to each other.

DISCUSSION QUESTIONS
FOR "THE GREAT COMMOTION: A LION STORY"

1. What was the problem in the story? (Bird and Snake were fighting.)
2. Why were they fighting? (They didn't like each other because they were different from each other.)
3. How did Lion and the other animals help Bird and Snake? (They stopped them from fighting and had them talk about how they were feeling.)
4. What did Lion say to them to help them? (You don't have to like everyone, but you have to be kind to each other.)
5. This is an opportunity to talk about the values of respect, kindness, and tolerance of others who are different than you.

PART II: PRIMARY ELEMENTARY STORIES

THE LOST BEAR

One day, Lion was walking around the woods, as lions do. All of the sudden he heard a strange noise. There, in the middle of the trees, was a Baby Bear, lying on his back and crying! Lion walked around the Baby Bear. He sniffed it, nudged it, and even licked it, but the Baby Bear would not stop crying. Lion didn't know what to do. He called out for his friend Bird to help him.

"Bird, I have found this Baby Bear crying in the woods. I don't know what to do to make him stop crying. Can you help me?"

Bird replied, "You have to pick the Baby up to make him stop crying. I can't pick him up because I will hurt him with my claws. Besides, the Baby is too big and heavy for me."

Lion said, "My paws are too big and rough to pick up a Baby. Maybe I can ask some of our other friends to help."

Lion called to Snake to ask for help. "Snake, I have found this Baby Bear crying in the woods. Bird said I should pick him up, but my paws are too big and rough. Can you help me?"

Snake said in his hissing voice, "I can't help you. I have no hands so I can't pick him up."

"Bird can't help me, Snake can't help me; what should I do now?" Lion thought to himself.

Just then, Lion saw Bunny hopping nearby. Lion called out to him, "Bunny, I have found this Baby Bear crying in the woods. Bird said I should pick him up, but my paws are too big and rough. Bird said his claws are too sharp, and Snake has no hands. Can you help me?"

"I'm sorry, Lion but I am just too small to help you. This Baby is bigger than me! I can't pick him up."

Lion was really worried. Baby Bear would not stop crying. Lion really wanted to help. He saw Frog hopping by, and called out to him. "Frog, I have found this Baby Bear crying in the woods. Bird said I should pick him up, but my paws are too big and rough, Bird said his claws are too sharp, Snake has no hands, and Bunny said she is too little. Can you help me?"

"I am too slippery and too small to pick him up," said Frog. "I wonder, though, if we all work together maybe we can help you pick up Baby Bear so he will stop crying."

"That is a great idea," said Lion. "Bird, Snake, Bunny, can you all help so we can pick up Baby Bear together?" Lion asked.

"Yes!" they all replied.

Snake slithered close to the Baby and circled him with his body, hugging him. The Baby began to quiet down. Bunny snuggled under the Baby's head to begin to lift him from the ground, and Frog hopped under his legs to help lift them from the ground. Lion was then able to gently reach under the Baby's head and legs to pick him up and hold him carefully against his heart. The beating of Lion's heart and the warmth of this body let the Baby relax, smile, and fall asleep. All the while, Bird had been circling overhead, looking for Mommy Bear.

"I found Mommy Bear," said Bird excitedly. "It looks like she has been searching for her Baby all this time. I will lead her to you."

When Mommy Bear arrived, she saw her Baby cuddled in Lion's arms, fast asleep. Lion was looking down at Baby Bear, smiling and happy. Snake, Bunny, and Frog were sitting in a circle around Lion and the Baby.

"Thank you all so much for taking such good care of my Baby. He was with me, and then I turned around and he was not there anymore. I was so worried. You have been great friends."

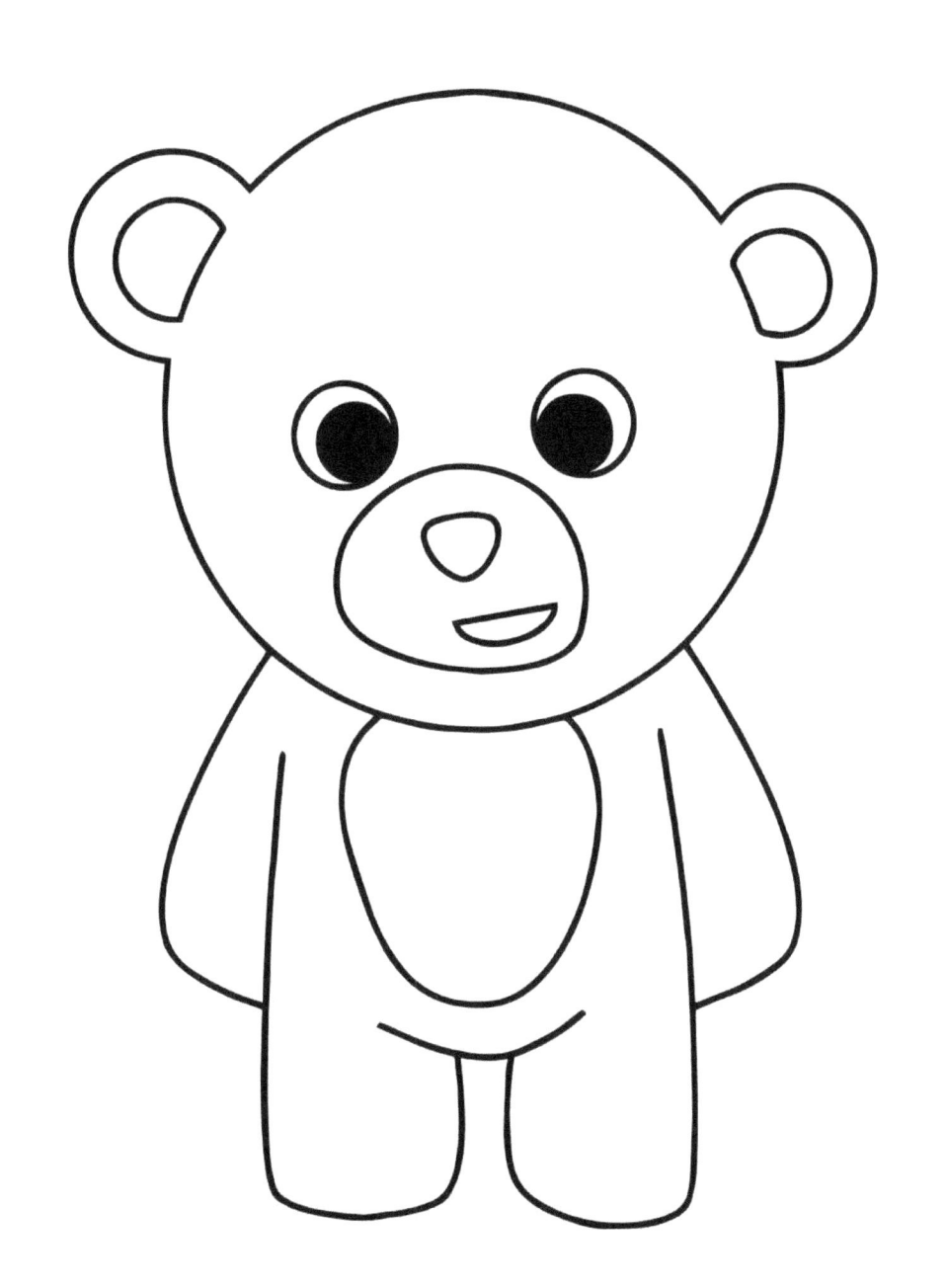

DISCUSSION QUESTIONS FOR "THE LOST BEAR"

1. What did Lion find in the woods?
2. Why do you think the Baby was crying?
3. Who came by to help? (Bird, Snake, Bunny, and Frog.)
4. How were they able to help the Baby? (They had to work together to pick the Baby up because each one alone could not do it by themselves.)
5. What happened when Bird found Mommy Bear? (Mommy was so happy to have found her Baby Bear and grateful that the animals had taken such good care of Baby Bear.)
6. What did the animals learn? (That when you work together with others you can do things that you might not be able to do by yourself.)

Part III:
INTERMEDIATE ELEMENTARY STORIES
(Third Grade - Fifth Grade)

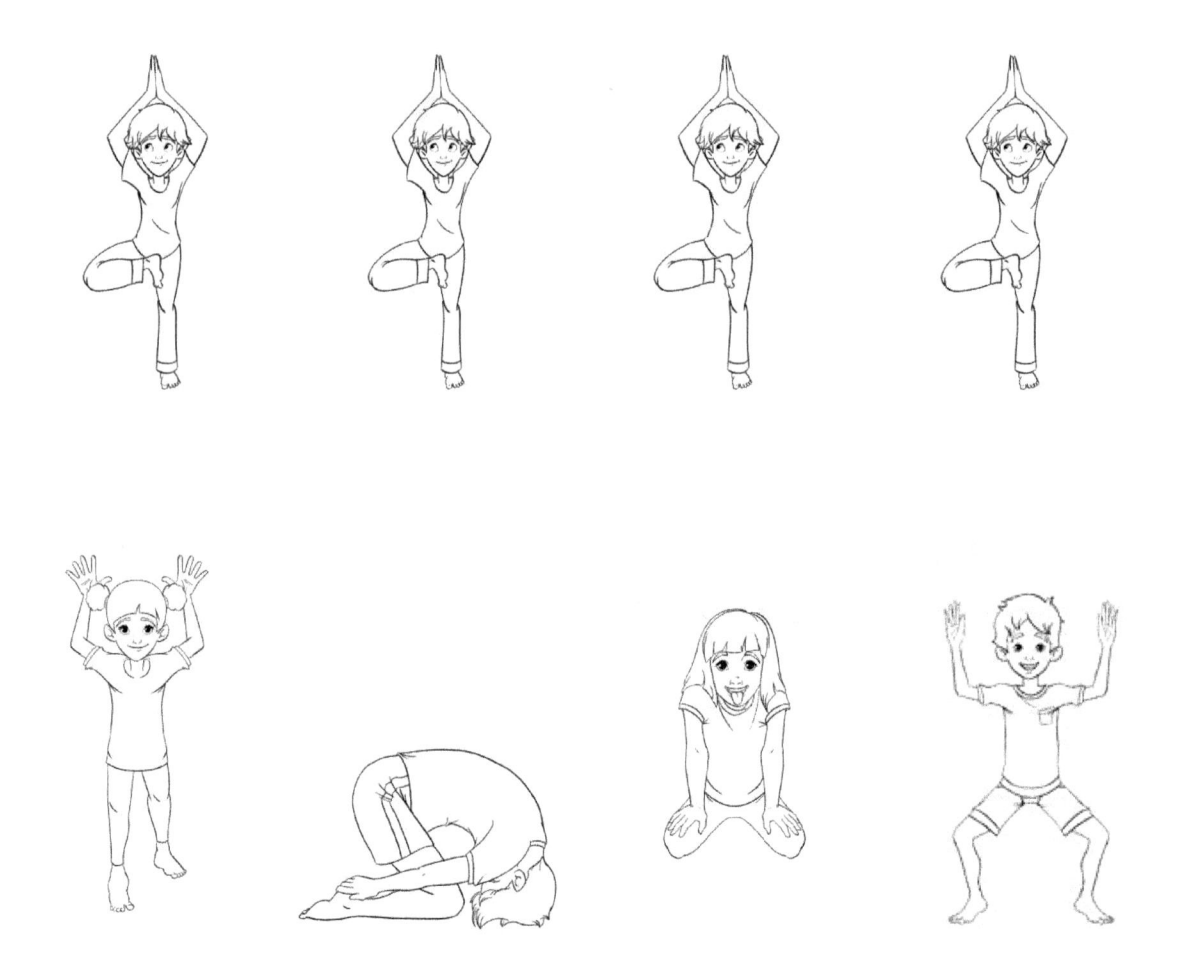

PART III: INTERMEDIATE ELEMENTARY STORIES

YOGA FOREST STORY

Once upon a time there was a forest deep in the woods.

There were many kinds of trees; some tall, some wide, some small, some with hanging arched branches, and some with branches pointing up. The trees would sway in the warm breeze throughout the day.

In this forest there was also a round, clear space in the center, where you could see the sun rise in the morning and set in the evening, and you could see the moon rise in the evening and set in the morning.

There were many animals in this forest: Bears, Deer, Rabbits, Turtles, Snails, Snakes, Horses, and Birds, including Eagles. They were all different.

But every morning at sunrise, and every evening at sundown, all the animals came together to the clearing in the forest. They stood side by side and watched the sun and the moon. They were friends with each other, even though they were different. They spent this time together, and then they went off into the forest to do whatever they had to do.

One day a new animal came into the forest. The animals had never seen any other animal like that one before. He was very large, bigger than any of the other animals in the forest. He looked down upon them and he had a large voice. The animals invited him to join them in their circle at the beginning and ending of each day. They didn't mind that he looked or sounded different. After all, they were all different from each other. When they asked him who he was, he replied, "I am a Surox. And, I am bigger than all of you." He then started to make fun of the Bears, Deer, Rabbits, Turtles, Snails, Snakes, Horses, and Birds. The animals didn't know what to do. They had never been made fun of before. They had always known that each one was different from the other, but they had always been friends anyway.

What would you do if you were the Bear, Deer, Rabbit, Turtle, Snail, Snake, Horse, or Bird?

The animals looked at each other and began to talk among themselves. They began to nod in agreement. Then, the littlest Bird said to the Surox, "We are happy with who we are and that we are all different. We are all friends. We would like to be friends with you too. We still invite you to be with us at sunrise and sunset. Will you be our friend?"

The Surox was surprised. No one had really wanted to be his friend before. Others had only made fun of him because he was so big and so different. He thought he should make fun of others first, because others would just make fun of him anyway. But now it seemed he had found a place where he could have friends.

He said, "I'm sorry I said those things to you. I would like to be a friend. I will join you at sunrise and sunset."

And he did! And everyone was happy.

DISCUSSION QUESTION
FOR "YOGA FOREST STORY"

1. How did the Surox act when he met the animals in the forest? What did he say to them? (He made fun of them.)
2. How did the animals feel when the Surox was talking to them? (They were confused. They had never been treated like that before.)
3. What did the animals say to the Surox? (They accepted him even though he was different. They invited him to be their friend.)
4. How did the Surox feel after the animals spoke to him? (Surprised) Why did he feel that way? (He was used to people making fun of him, so he made fun of others).
5. What happened at the end of the story? (The Surox and the other animals made friends.)

6. This is an opportunity to talk about bullying and how important it is to be kind to others even though we may be different and have different experiences than they.

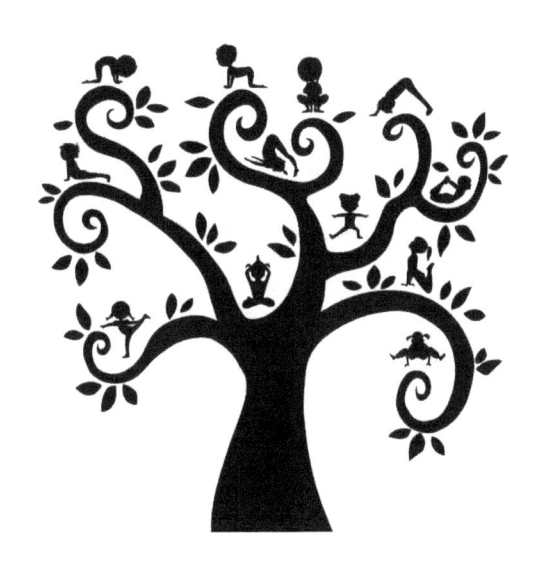

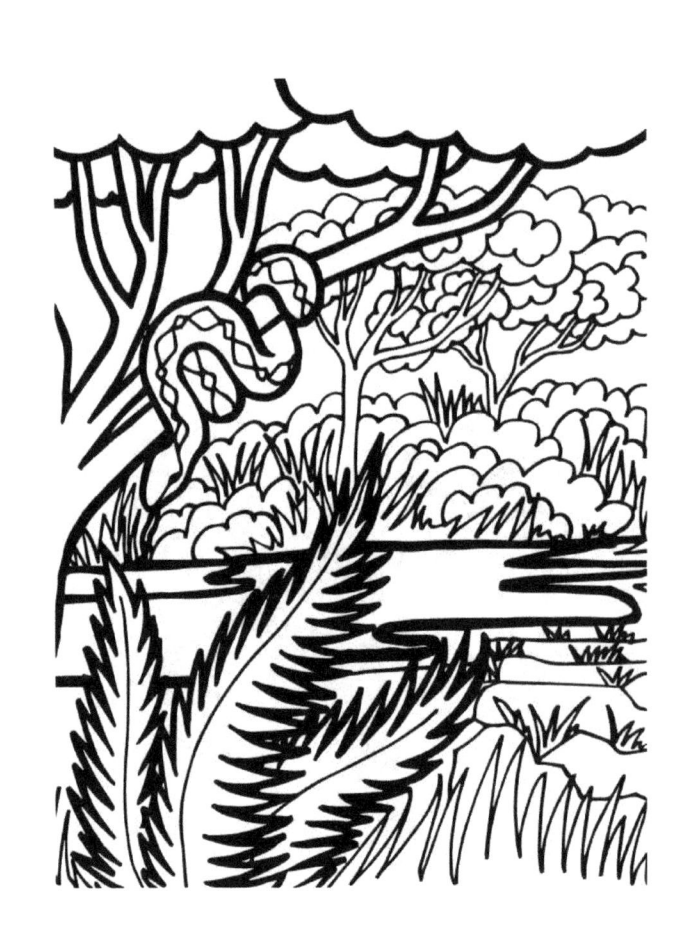

PART III: INTERMEDIATE ELEMENTARY STORIES

JUNGLE STORY

Sue and Tom lived in a small house with their parents at the edge of a jungle. From their house they could often hear strange noises from the jungle: the loud caw of a bird, the deep roar of a lion, chattering and laughing of monkeys, the snaps and crackles of branches of trees, the rustling of leaves in the breeze, the hoot of owls, as well as noises that they could not recognize like whistles and cries that were sometimes scary. Their Mom and Dad told them not to go into the jungle because it could be dangerous.

Sue and Tom had a cat named Nellie. Nellie lived in the house and never went outside. The jungle could be dangerous for Nellie too! But one day Nellie got out of the house, and after hearing a loud screeching sound, Nellie ran into the jungle! Sue and Tom were scared for Nellie. Their Mom and Dad were not home. They didn't know what to do! They knew they were not supposed to go into the jungle, but they had to find her. So, they decided they just had to go into the jungle to look for her.

Sue and Tom crept along on tiptoe, looking for Nellie while trying not to run into any of the animals they heard. They climbed over fallen branches and under big thick plants with wide leaves that were as tall as their heads. They saw snakes slithering down trees, big yellow and green frogs leaping out from under bushes, and birds flying overhead.

But – all of the sudden – something strange happened. The frogs started to roar like a lion, the snakes started to caw like a bird, and the birds started to laugh like a monkey! They looked at each other with surprise. They could not believe it. "What is happening here?" they asked together. They had to go on to look for Nellie, so they went deeper into the jungle. They crossed over a stream and saw water bubbling over rocks in the winding shallow stream bed. They saw small and large fish darting through the water. Some of the fish began to jump out of the water and land back in with a splash. They thought they heard an owl hooting in the trees above the stream, but when they looked up they saw a leopard sitting in the branches looking at them. They were sure the leopard was going to jump down and run after them, but instead it blinked sleepily and began to make a hooting sound. There was no owl; it was a leopard all along! Then they heard a whistle coming from the stream and they looked down quickly. The fish that were jumping out of the water began to whistle as they jumped! None of this was what they expected.

"What kind of place is this?" they asked. They still had not found Nellie, so they decided to go a little further. The trees were harder to climb through because there were so many of them. There were long branches that fell from the top of the trees to the ground that they had to sweep out of the way to get through to the other side. They heard the sounds of crickets, but were unsure if they were really crickets or some other creature they had not yet seen. Finally, they reached a clearing in the trees and you won't believe what they saw. There was a mouse sitting on top of a huge elephant, and Nellie was lying in the sun at the elephant's feet, cleaning her paws! Nellie looked up when she saw Sue and Tom, jumped to her feet and happily trotted over to them.

"Oh Nellie," they said, "We are so glad to see you! We are going to take you home." Nellie purred and snuggled in their arms.

As they turned away from the clearing to go back through the jungle to their home, they heard two more sounds. They turned around and, believe it or not, the mouse was screeching loudly, and the elephant was crying softly. Sue and Tom looked at each other. "I guess they are going to miss Nellie," they said.

They turned around and walked home. This was certainly a day that was filled with unexpected things.

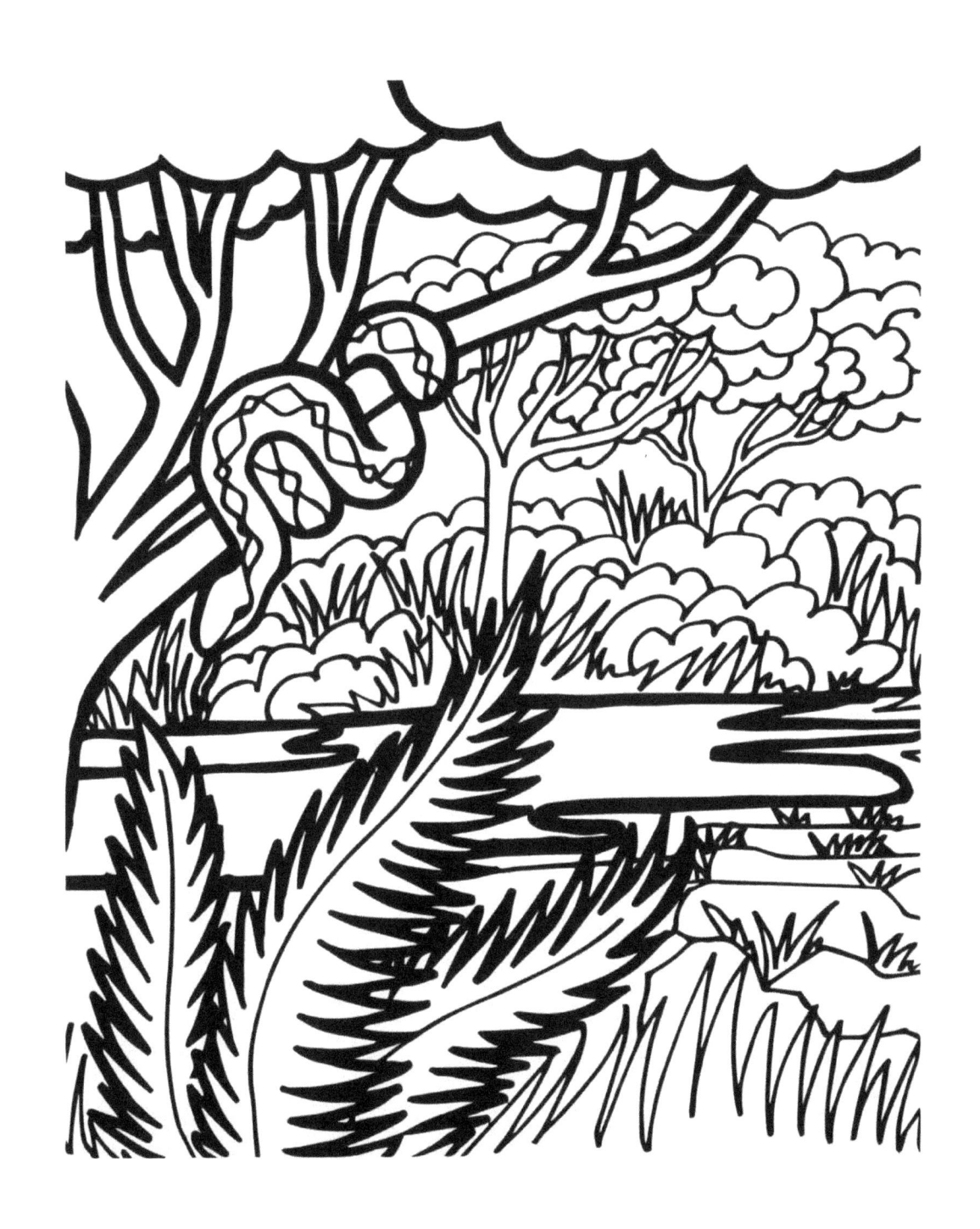

DISCUSSION QUESTIONS FOR "JUNGLE STORY"

1. Why do you think Tom's and Sue's mother and father told them not to go into the woods? (It could be dangerous.)
2. Why do you think they went out to look for Nellie? (They were scared for her.)
3. What did they see and hear when they went into the woods? (Noises, from animals, unusual and unexpected.)
4. Were Tom and Sue brave? Why? (They searched for Nellie even though they saw and heard unexpected things.)
5. This is an opportunity to discuss the concept of pursuing a goal even when unexpected things happen.

PART III: INTERMEDIATE ELEMENTARY STORIES

THANKSGIVING

There was once a great warrior. His name was Sun Ray. He had a sister, Moon Beam, who was known far and wide for her great skills.

From the time they were small children, about the age you are now, they learned to use a bow and arrow. They learned to shoot long and straight.

They learned when to be still and when to move.

They learned to move quietly, with control, while going slow as well as fast.

They ran quietly and swiftly as deer. They could be as quiet and small as a mouse.

One fall day, just before Thanksgiving, they were given the job of finding a wild turkey. The turkeys were rare in their land.

Sun Ray and Moon Beam had to go search for them in the fields, and then in the forest. They had to be quiet, so that they could listen for the sound of the turkeys as they walked over the leaves and made soft breath sounds with their beaks and tiny crunch sounds with their feet. Sun Ray and Moon Beam walked and searched for many hours. They saw:

    Eagles fly overhead,
    Turtles on the ground,
    Snakes climbing the trees, and
    Rabbits in the woods.

Finally, they found a turkey. Quietly they raised their bow and arrow. They looked carefully. The turkey was so beautiful and peaceful. They did not want to harm it. They watched the turkey for a while, and thought carefully about the right thing to do. A great warrior has to stop and think, make decisions, and stay in control. They looked at each other, speaking to each other with their eyes. They nodded silently, and then slowly began to back away from the turkey and head home. On the way home, they found potatoes and vegetables and wheat. They gathered as much as their arms could carry and when they got home they made a delicious meal from all that they had. They had a very happy Thanksgiving.

DISCUSSION QUESTIONS FOR "THANKSGIVING"

1. What does the story tell us about what it takes to be a great warrior? (A great warrior has to be able to stop and think, make decisions, and stay in control.)
2. Were Sun Ray and Moon Beam great warriors? Why? (They knew when to be still and when to move. They could move quietly with control when they were going fast and slow. They were able to control their body movement. They were patient.)
3. How did Sun Ray and Moon Beam talk to each other without using words? (They spoke to each other with their eyes and by nodding their heads.)
4. What decision did they make about the turkey? Why do you think they made that decision? (They chose to let the turkey go free. They thought it was beautiful and peaceful. They did not want to harm it.)
5. Did they have enough food for Thanksgiving? What did they find to eat? (They found plenty of potatoes, and vegetables, and wheat to make bread.)

PART III: INTERMEDIATE ELEMENTARY STORIES

HOMER'S EMERGENCY

Homer always complained. When the sun was out it was too bright. When the rain came it was too dark. When it was summer it was too hot, and when it was winter it was too cold. Not only that – when he complained, he REALLY complained! His problems were always the worst, bigger and more terrible than anyone else's problems.

One morning, as Homer was getting ready for school, his nose began to twitch and all of the sudden he sneezed.

"Mom," he yelled. "Mom, come quick. It's an emergency!"

Mom rushed up the stairs and ran into his room. "Homer, what's wrong?" she cried.

"Mom, I'm sick! I sneezed!!!" Homer responded.

"Oh," said Mom. "Well, do you feel like you have to sneeze again?"

"No," Homer responded, "but I'm sure it will happen again. I am sick. I might have the flu, or even pneumonia!"

"Well, let me check your temperature," said Mom. She took out a thermometer, put it under his tongue, and waited. "No, your temperature is normal," she said. "Perhaps it was just dust. I think you are OK. Time to get ready for school."

Homer sighed and slowly got up. He was sure he was terribly sick, and Mom didn't believe him. He would have to go to school, but he just knew he would be in the hospital soon.

When he got to school he walked into his classroom with his head down, his shoulders slumped, and his steps heavy. He slowly put his things away and walked over to his desk, and he put his head down on his arms. His teacher came by to hand out morning work.

"What's the matter Homer? Are you tired today?" she asked.

"I'm sick, Mrs. B. I sneezed this morning. I might have the flu or even worse," replied Homer.

"Well, let's see how you do for a while. If you need to you can see the nurse a little later."

Homer looked up at her sadly and nodded.

Homer got through his morning. He didn't sneeze again, but he remained sure he was really sick. When it was time for recess, Mrs. B said, "Homer, if you still feel you are sick, you can go see the nurse now."

Homer didn't feel like playing, so he slowly shuffled down the hall to the nurse's office. When he got there, the nurse was sitting at her desk.

"Hello Homer," the nurse said. "How are you today?"

"I'm sick," Homer replied. "Very sick. I'm sure I have the flu, or even worse, maybe pneumonia."

"What makes you think that?" asked the nurse.

"I sneezed this morning. I just know I am sick," said Homer.

"Well, let's check you out and see," said the nurse. She took out her thermometer and checked his temperature. "Normal," she said. "Let's look at your eyes, ears, and throat. Humm, all looking good." She felt his neck, listened to his heart and lungs, and then said, "Everything looks good."

"Are you sure I'm not sick?" Homer asked.

"I'm sure," said the nurse. "Do you feel a little better now?"

"I guess so. I'm starting to," said Homer.

"Great. Here are some things you can do if you start to get worried or don't feel quite right. Let's try them together:"

The nurse taught Homer three different ways to breathe, to help him to calm down: Belly Breath, "Count to Five" Breath, and Alternate Nostril Breath. Then she taught him three balancing poses to help him feel steady and in control: Tree (Vriksasana), Bird (Virabhadrasana), and Eagle (Garudasana).

"How do you feel now, Homer?" asked the nurse.

"I feel a lot better now," said Homer. "Thanks!"

"I'm so glad," said the nurse with a big smile. "Now go back to class and enjoy your day."

So, Homer went back to class. He did not sneeze again for the rest of the day. He did his work, ate lunch, and played with his friends. When he got home, his Mom asked him how his day went.

"It was OK," said Homer.

"And how are you feeling?" asked Mom.

"I am OK. I thought I was really sick, but I guess you can sneeze sometimes without it being a big problem. And the nurse showed me some things to do when I get worried or I don't feel right. Want to see?"

"Sure," said Mom. Homer showed his Mom the breathing and balances that made him feel better.

"That's great," said his Mom. "Now you know some things that can help you feel better. Let's try to keep that in mind for next time."

"I will, Mom," said Homer.

DISCUSSION QUESTIONS FOR "HOMER'S PROBLEM"

1. Why did Homer think he was sick? (He sneezed.)
2. Did Homer think he had a big problem? (Yes.)
3. What did the nurse do to make Homer feel better? (She took his temperature and checked him, and then taught him how to breathe to help him feel better when he got worried.)
4. Did Homer feel better? (Yes.)
5. What did Homer learn? (That not all problems are "big" problems and that breathing will help him calm down.)

These are the **Breathing Strategies** Homer learned:

Alternate Nostril Breathing:

Using your right hand, close the right nostril with the thumb. Fold the index and middle finger down toward the palm, and place the ring finger to the side of the left nostril. Breath in through the left nostril while holding the right side closed, hold the breath for a count of four, then place the ring finger over the left nostril while releasing the right thumb and allowing the breath to exhale out of the right nostril. Hold the hand in place, and breathe into the right nostril, again holding the breath for a count of four, then release the ring finger from the left nostril while covering the right nostril with the thumb while exhaling out of the left side. Repeat this process for a cycle of eight times.

"Count to Five" Breath:

Hold the right hand in front of the face with all five fingers open. Blow out on each finger as if you are blowing out a candle.

Belly Breath:

Breathe deeply into the belly, feeling it expand on the inhale and contract on the exhale. Repeat four times.

PART III: INTERMEDIATE ELEMENTARY STORIES

COPYING AND TEASING

James and Sam were friends, well at least sometimes they were friends. They went to the same school and were in the same class. They sat near each other, so they could see each other in the classroom.

Sometimes they played nicely with each other. They liked the same games and could take turns playing.

Sometimes James would copy what Sam was saying and doing. That made Sam mad.

Sometimes when the teacher gave a direction, Sam would say the same direction to James. That made James mad.

When James copied Sam, and Sam told James what to do, they would yell at each other.

The teacher had to make sure that they were not near each other so that James and Sam could calm down.

How could James and Sam solve this problem? They wanted to be friends but they really made each other angry.

The teacher talked with James and Sam.

"Sam," she said, "why do you get angry at James?"

"I get mad at James because he copies what I say. I don't like that. It feels like he is teasing me," said Sam.

"James," said the teacher, "are you trying to tease Sam?"

"No," said James. "I can't always stop myself. When I hear something, I just say it. I'm sorry."

"James, why do you get angry at Sam?" asked the teacher.

"I get mad at Sam because he tells me what to do. I already know what to do because you told me. I don't need to hear it again," said James.

"Sam, are you trying to make James angry?"

"No," said Sam. "When I see that someone is not doing what you say, I say it again, just in case they didn't hear me. I am not trying to make James angry."

"So, both of you repeat what you hear, right?" said the teacher.

"Yes," they said together.

Sam and James looked at each other.

They learned that they were not trying to make the other person angry, but they both repeated things that they heard!

"We may not be able to stop repeating things we hear, but we can try not to get angry about it," said Sam.

"Yeah," said James, "we can try that."

"I can help you remember that you are not trying to make each other angry," said the teacher.

"It's a deal," said Sam and James together.

They smiled.

DISCUSSION QUESTIONS FOR "COPYING AND TEASING"

1. Why did Sam and James get angry at each other? (James would copy whatever Sam was saying, and Sam would repeat teacher directions to James.)
2. What did Sam tell the teacher about why he was angry at James? (Sam said it felt like James was teasing him.)
3. What did James tell the teacher about why he was angry at Sam? (James felt that Sam was always telling him what to do, when he already heard the directions from the teacher.)
4. Did Sam and James want to make each other angry? (No.)

5. What did they learn about each other? (They both repeated things that they heard. They wanted to be friends but they could not stop repeating what they heard.)
6. How did they solve their problem? (They made a deal to help each other remember that they were not trying to make the other angry, but they had a hard time not repeating what they heard.)
7. This can be used as an opportunity to talk about understanding each other and coping with differences.

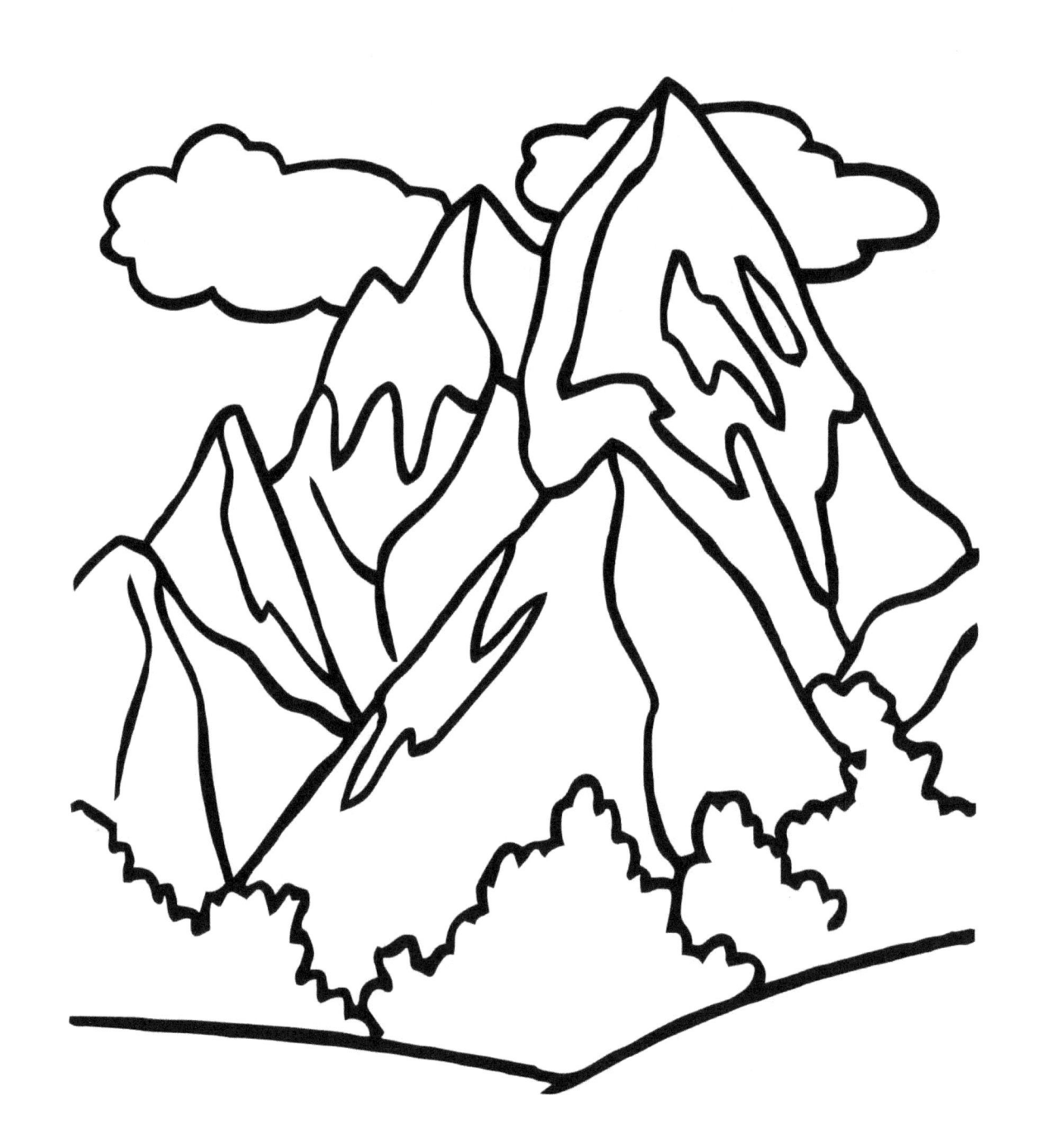

PART III: INTERMEDIATE ELEMENTARY STORIES

THE MOUNTAIN CLIMB

There was once a very tall mountain far, far away. From a distance, it looked like the mountain was hanging in the sky. The mountain was so tall that the clouds covered the top most of the time. Every now and then, if you were really lucky, you could see the top. If you looked very closely, the top seemed to glow with a red light.

Very few people had ever been able to climb to the top of the mountain. Those people who had done it said that there were really five levels from the bottom to the top, and each level was very different.

One day, a boy named Salmi decided he wanted to try to reach the top of the mountain. He was a boy about your age. He asked his friend Reva, a girl from his town, if she would go with him. Salmi and Riva had helped each other go through many adventures.

Early in the morning, when the sun rose, they set off on their journey. They walked many miles, through tall grass, muddy river beds, and under low hanging branches of trees on their way. After a long time, they finally made it to the foot of the mountain. There were small rocks and large boulders all around them. There were also long flat rocks, and flowers, and bushes between the rocks, and butterflies resting on top. They sat down to rest on one of the long flat rocks, had some water and food that they brought with them, and took a deep breath to get ready for their climb. They looked up, and saw that there were clouds hanging over the mountain, so they could not see very far. They knew they were on the first level, at the bottom of the mountain, and they thought they could see the next level, but they were not quite sure. Even so, they decided that they felt happy and calm and they were ready to move on.

They began to climb. It was like going up a hill that was made of rocks and earth. They began to feel the muscles in their legs work, but it was not hard. They saw some squirrels looking for food. They found lizards sitting on rocks that ran away when they got close. When Salmi and Reva looked up they saw that they still had a long way to go, so they were a little concerned but they were still calm. After a while they reached a ledge on the rock, and they stopped to rest and drink water. They had finished the second level.

Salmi and Reva looked up the mountain, and saw that the climb to the next level would be harder. There was no more dirt around them and the rocks were higher. They looked at each other and took a deep breath. They were a little worried, but they knew they could help each other if they needed to. They began to climb. Their leg muscles were really working now. They saw some mountain goats leap from rock to rock. They also saw some snakes slither over the rock and disappear in the cracks between them. They were getting closer to the clouds that were hanging over the mountain. The weather had been warm, but it was turning cooler now that they were climbing higher. After a long time, they reached a rock that had a ledge where they could sit and rest. They had reached the third level. They were tired and worried. They took a breath, had some water, and talked.

"Salmi, are you sure you want to go on?" asked Reva. "The rocks ahead are higher and steeper."

"Yes, Reva," Salmi replied. "I want to see the top of the mountain. I know we can do it."

Salmi and Reva began to climb. They needed to use their hands to pull them up the rocks while they pressed down with their legs. It was very hard work. They had to move more slowly, and they had to help each other. Salmi or Reva would climb up a steep rock, and then turn to help the other climb up before they could move on. Around the side of the mountain they saw mountain lions sleeping on the rocks. They had to be quiet so they would not wake the mountain lions. They also saw birds circling around the mountain, their wings spread wide as they glided in the air. It was colder now, and it was harder to breathe. They had to take their time and move carefully.

Finally, after what felt like a long time, they reached a ledge in the rocks where they could stop to rest. They took a deep breath and had some water. They had finished the fourth level. They were in the clouds. It was cold and damp. They could not see very far around them. They were scared but they wanted to get to the top. They looked at each other.

"Salmi, I am really tired and scared," Reva said. "Do you really think we can make it to the top?"

Salmi replied, "I am scared too, but we have each other. I know we can do it. Let's rest a little more, and think about how good it will be to finish, and how we can help each other. Being scared will make us more careful, but it doesn't have to stop us."

Reva nodded. They rested until they were sure they were ready to go on.

They then began the final climb. This time it was harder than ever before. Some of the rocks went straight up! They had to pull with their arms, push with their legs, and find ways around rocks that were just too hard, even though they were helping each other. It was really cold. There was even some snow on the rocks! They heard birds around them, but they could not see them because of the clouds.

They were scared, but they kept on trying, one step at a time. They took deep breaths, moved slowly, stopped when they needed to rest, and talked to each other to figure out what step they would take next.

They worked hard. Finally, they climbed above the clouds! Just a little more and they would be at the top! They were really tired, but happy that they were almost there, even though it was so hard. They could see a red glow just above them. They could now see the birds above them. They pulled and pushed and breathed, and pulled and pushed some more.

At last they were at the top. They had made it to the fifth level. They were so happy. They could see the red rim at the top of the mountain. All the sudden they realized that it was a volcano! They looked down, and they could see red lava deep below. What should they do now?

Salmi and Reva froze in place. They were scared.

What if the volcano erupted?

They looked at each other. Their bodies felt tense. They took a deep breath to calm down. They talked, and thought, and then decided that they needed to move slowly and calmly so that they would stay safe. So Salmi and Reva began slowly to go down the mountain, step by step, level by level, moving quietly, slowly, carefully, helping each other and taking one deep breath at a time. But as they began to climb down, they looked out over the land below.

It was beautiful! They saw valleys, and grasses, and waterfalls, and animals, and an eagle soaring, and far below, their very own town. Even though it was hard work to climb the mountain, and scary too, they were happy that they made the journey. Now they knew that they could do something hard and scary and they would be ok. They would see new things and learn new things, and that made them feel happy and proud.

DISCUSSION QUESTIONS FOR "THE MOUNTAIN CLIMB"

1. How many levels did Salmi and Reva have to climb to get to their goal, the top of the mountain? (Five.)
2. How did they feel at each level? What strategies did they use at each level to help them continue to their goal?
   @ Level 1: Salmi and Reva were happy and calm and ready to move on.
   @ Level 2: Salmi and Reva were a little concerned, but still calm. They rested until they were ready to move on.
   @ Level 3: They were tired and worried, but still focused on their goal. They rested until they were ready to move on.

*@ **Level 4***: They were tired and scared. They rested longer and talked about helping each other through the difficult journey.

*@ **Level 5***: They were scared. They had to move slowly one step at a time. They had to work together to move forward safely. They were happy that they made it, and then scared when they made their discovery.

3. What coping strategies did they use to help them after they reached the top of the mountain? (They remained calm so they could think clearly about what to do. They took deep breaths. They moved carefully so they would stay safe.)
4. Were Salmi and Reva happy that they made the journey? Why? (They were happy they accomplished something that was hard for them.)
5. This can be an opportunity for the children to discuss how they coped with things that were hard for them.

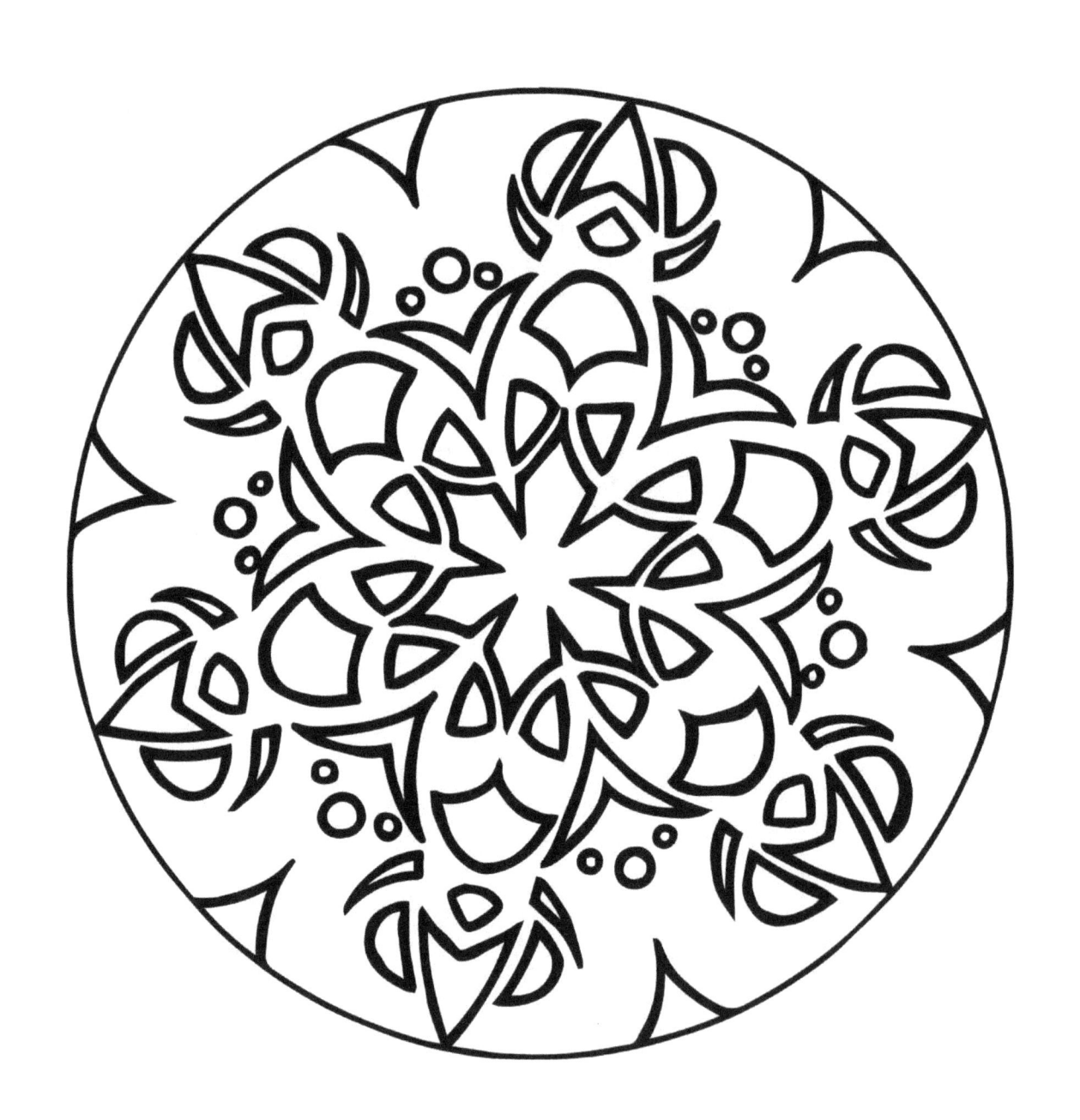

PART III: INTERMEDIATE ELEMENTARY STORIES

THE SEED INSIDE

Mara was 8 years old. She lived with her Grandma. She didn't know where her Mom and Dad were, or if they would be back. Mara was angry. When she went to school she was angry. When kids tried to play with her she was angry. When her teacher said she was doing a good job she was angry. She just couldn't help herself. She felt like there was a soda bottle inside her that was always fizzing angry, and that it would pop at any moment.

Mara's Grandma kept on telling her she had a seed inside her, a seed of goodness that was who she was. She could let the seed grow, or she could hold it back from growing. Being angry held the seed back. Mara wanted to believe her Grandma, but she just couldn't help herself.

"You know, Mara, when you feel that soda bottle fizzing in your belly, take a breath, tighten your body, and then let it go. It can help to keep a cap on that bottle inside you, so that your seed can grow," Grandma said.

The next day Mara went to school. She decided she would try to do what her Grandma said the next time she felt angry. Sure enough, a kid in her class started to complain about something and make a lot of noise. Mara felt that soda fizzing inside her again. The fizzing got bigger and bigger and was about to pop. Mara tried to take a breath, but she just couldn't make it happen. She was angry, and now she felt disappointed too. She felt she had let her Grandma down. She stayed angry all day. It is better to be angry then sad, she thought to herself. People will stay away from me then and I won't have to feel sad anymore.

When she got home, Grandma asked her how her day went.

Mara was too sorry that she couldn't do what her Grandma had asked her to do, so she said, "Everyone was just bothering me today. I'm just angry."

Grandma said, "Maybe tomorrow will be better. Remember you have that seed of goodness in you. It will come out, I'm sure of it." Mara was surprised.

Grandma didn't seem mad at her. Mara decided that she would try again tomorrow to do that breath thing.

When Mara got to school the next day, she had in her mind that she was going to take that breath, tighten and release her body, and feel better. She felt a little tickle inside her when she thought about it. Maybe that seed of goodness is starting to grow, she thought. But at math class the teacher said they were going to have a test today. Mara knew that she had missed some of the math lessons. Because she had been so angry, she just couldn't listen to the teacher. She knew she was not going to do well on the test, and she started to feel anxious. Then she thought that it's better to feel angry than anxious, so she burst out loud, "I'm not taking any test!" She began to think that it was everyone else's fault that she didn't know the math, because they had made her angry.

The teacher had Mara take the test in the hallway, because she was making too much noise in class. She stayed angry all day. When she got home, Grandma asked her how her day went today.

"I was angry because I had to take a math test today," Mara replied. Mara really felt sorry though.

Grandma said, "Well, sometimes school is hard, but I know you can do it. Remember, you have that seed of goodness inside. Tomorrow may be a better day."

Mara was surprised again. Grandma wasn't mad. She still believed in her! Mara decided she would try again tomorrow. She liked it when she felt the seed of goodness stir inside her. Maybe she could make that happen again.

The next day, Mara returned to school, ready to try. In math, the teacher returned the math test. Mara didn't do great, but she didn't do so badly either. She felt relieved, and she felt the seed of goodness start to stir. That kid in class began to complain again. He didn't do so great on the math test. Mara looked up and started to feel the soda bubbles inside, but she caught herself. She took a breath, tightened her muscles, and felt the soda bubbles stop. Then she let the breath go.

She thought she felt the seed grow a little bigger! The teacher caught her eye and smiled at her!

"Wow, I did it!" she thought.

Later in the day, another kid started to get on her nerves. She thought the kid was laughing at her. She felt the soda bubbles start to fizz. She looked around and saw that another kid was doing some crazy dance moves across the room. She took a breath, tightened her muscles, and let her breath go. The kid that was laughing wasn't laughing at her, but at the kid with the crazy dance moves!

The seed inside her grew a little more. She got through the day and was able to hold back her anger two times! When she got home, Grandma asked her how her day went.

Mara said, "You know, it went pretty well today!"

Grandma smiled. Her eyes twinkled. "I have a feeling that that seed of goodness inside you grew today," she said.

Mara replied, "You know, Grandma, I think you might be right."

DISCUSSION QUESTIONS FOR "THE SEED INSIDE"

1. Have you ever felt like Mara?
2. What kind of things makes you angry?
3. Where do you feel it in your body?
4. Why do you feel that taking a breath and tightening muscles helped Mara calm down?
5. Let's practice that breath together, so that we can use it when we feel angry.

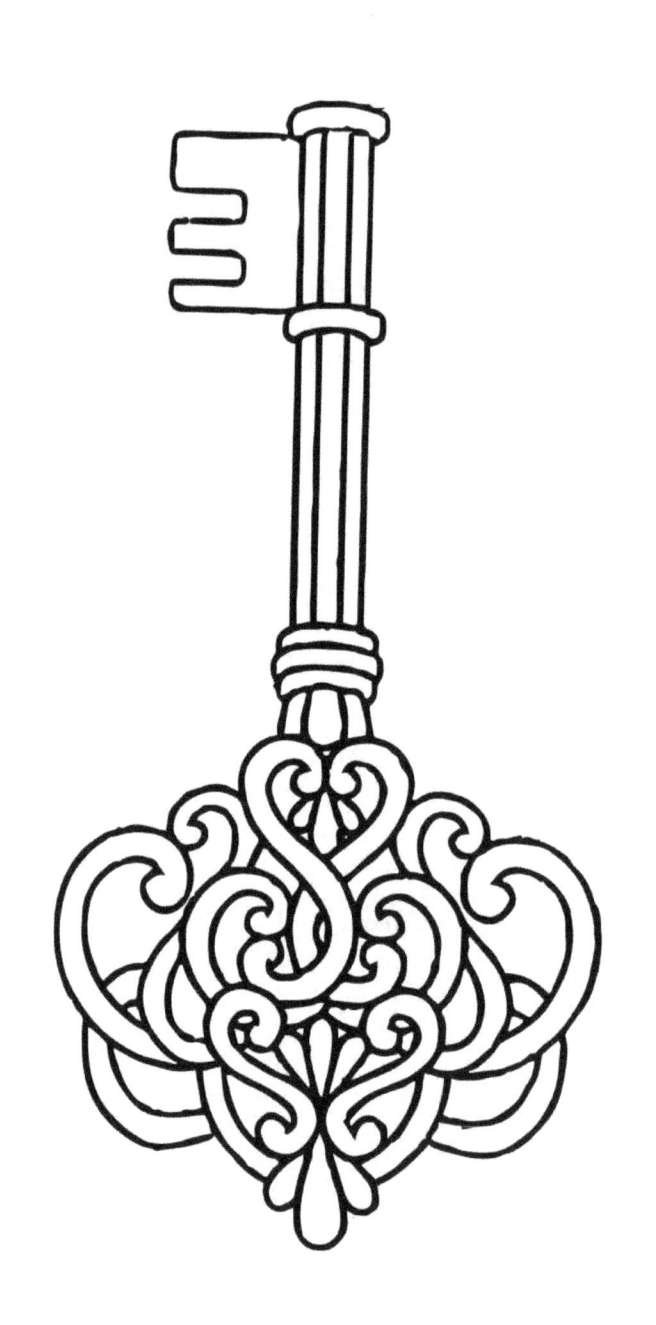

PART III: INTERMEDIATE ELEMENTARY STORIES

THE GATE

In the neighborhood, not far from the trees, there is a gate. Around the gate are stone walls that are tall, thick, and weathered gray. The gate itself is made of iron that is curled into patterns of leaves and flowers. Just inside the gate are thick vines that are twined together so that you can see pinpricks of light between the branches but you can't see what is beyond them. The vines reach way above the stone walls. In the middle of the gate there is a lock. The lock has an opening for a key, but it must be a really old key because I have never seen a lock like that one before. It doesn't look like that gate has been opened for a long time.

People pass that gate and stone wall all the time. It looks like a lot of people don't even notice it anymore. I got curious about it though, and I began to ask around about it. My Mom said that gate has been there as long as she could remember. She told me to ask the lady down the street, who lived in the neighborhood when she was little.

That lady, Mrs. K., had deep wrinkles in her face, gray hair that she wore in a tight bun, and thick glasses. She was short and her back was rounded and she always wore a sweater. She needed a cane to help her walk. I went to her house and asked her about the gate.

She said, "I know that gate. It was here when I was a child. I never saw anyone going in or out of that gate. You might want to ask Mr. Oden. He used to be a locksmith, like his Daddy before him. He still sits in his old shop, even though he doesn't work anymore. His grandson runs the business now. You seem like a kind boy. I think he would talk to you."

I got busy with school and stuff, and helping my Mom in the house, and I didn't get around to visiting Mr. Oden. I mentioned the gate to a few people I knew at school, though. Some of them hadn't noticed it at all. Some of them said they would try to climb it or force it to open, but I think they were just saying that. But that gate stayed in the back of my mind. One Saturday I had nothing else to do after I finished the stuff my Mom wanted me to do, so I decided to go to the locksmith shop to see if I could find out any more about the gate. The shop looked kind of dark and old. I asked the man at the counter if I could see Mr. Oden.

"He doesn't get many visitors anymore," said the man.

"I just wanted to ask him about an old gate," I replied. "Mrs. K sent me."

"In that case, come on back," said the man. "Grandpa, there's a young man here to see you about a gate! He knows Mrs. K."

I was led to a back room, where a really old man sat on a stool at an old wooden table, unlocking old locks with keys. His eyes looked huge behind his glasses. His head was bald except for a few wisps of hair sticking straight up in the air. His shoulders were rounded and he looked shrunken behind the wooden table.

"Hello, young man. You're a friend of Mrs. K? I haven't seen her in a long time. How can I help you?"

"There is an old gate with a big lock in the middle of a stone wall I have been curious about. Do you know what is behind it? Do you have a key that could open it? I have never seen anyone go in or out of it."

"I know that gate," said Mr. Oden. "It has been closed for a very long time. Way back, when the owner gave the key to my father, he said that it would take someone really special to be able to open it again. That man went away and no one ever saw him again."

"Do you still have that key? I would love to open the gate."

"I have the key, but the gate will not open for just anyone, even with the key. A few have tried it in the past, but no one has ever been able to open it. Maybe you will be the one to do it," said Mr. Oden.

Mr. Oden gave me the key. It was big and heavy, made of iron just like the gate. I was excited, and I thanked him and told him I would come back to let him know what happened.

The next day I took the key with me to school. I had it in my pocket and it really weighed me down. I showed the key to a few of my friends, and while I was doing that some other kids saw it.

"What ya got there?" said Von. Von was a big guy with a loud voice. He always seemed angry. I could hear him yell sometimes, and his classroom was down the hall from mine. He always had a few friends with him wherever he went.

"Just a key," I said.

"Is that a key to that gate I heard you were talking about? I'll take it, I'm sure I can open the gate." He grabbed the key out of my hand. He said, "If you want to watch me open it, meet me at the front steps after school. I'll be there with my guys, and we will head over there. Don't be late. I won't wait for you."

I had to get the key back, but he was too angry and strong for me to take it from him, so I knew I had to meet him after school. I decided to take my friend, Tai, with me so I could have someone to help me if things went sour.

After school, Tai and I ran to the front steps. We saw Von with a bunch of his friends just starting to walk in the direction of the gate when we got there.

"Told you, I wouldn't wait," said Von. "Keep up or lose!"

It wasn't too long before we got to the gate. Some of Von's friends said they never noticed it before. They were laughing and saying that the lock doesn't look like a big deal.

"Just watch this," said Von. He put the key in the lock. It wouldn't turn. He tried hitting it, pushing it, jiggling it, but it wouldn't budge.

"This is stupid. You got the wrong key," he said with anger. "If I can't open it, no one can." Von threw the key on the ground.

"Let me try," said Carl, one of his friends. Carl always wanted to do what Von did, and he always wanted what Von had. He grabbed the key and put it in the lock. He used both hands to try to turn it, but it would not budge.

"Yeah, this is stupid. You must be playing a trick on us," said Carl.

"I got it, I got it," said Tray, another of Von's friends. Tray was always buzzing about, moving and getting in everyone's way. Tray grabbed the key from Carl and started to shove it in the lock. He squirmed and jumped and jiggled, but the lock would not open.

"We're outa' here," said Von. "You just don't know what you are talking about with this key. You better not mess with me anymore or you will wish you hadn't," he said.

And with that, Von and his friends left the gate and walked away.

The key was still in the lock.

"Mr. Oden wouldn't give me the key if it was not the right one. He said that it would take someone special to open the lock. Maybe those guys just weren't it!" I said to Tai.

"Why don't you try it," said Tai.

I turned toward the lock. I thought about the people I had spent time with on this adventure, Mrs. K and Mr. Oden. I thought about how long the gate had been closed, and about my Mom, and even about my friend Tai. Even if I couldn't open the lock, I liked the time I spent with all of them and I was glad this adventure happened.

I slowly tried to turn the key, and I heard a click! The lock gave way and the gate opened.

DISCUSSION QUESTIONS FOR "THE GATE"

1. What was the value shown by the main character that allowed him to open the gate? (Kindness.)
2. How did he show that value in the story? (He showed by the way he treated others in the story.)

3. Did other characters in the story show that value? (Yes – Mrs. K, Mr. Oden, and Tai.)
4. Why didn't the key work for Von? (Because Von was not kind. He was always angry. He bullied others.)
5. Introduce the Yama principle of Ahimsa (Kindness). Talk about how that principle is present in this story.
   In the philosophy of Yoga, there are 10 principles for ways to live in the world. The first five are called Yamas, and they suggest how to live in society. The second ones are Niyamas, and they suggest how to become the best person we can be. The first Yama is called Ahimsa, which, means non-harming, and relates to being kind to others, as well as to ourselves.

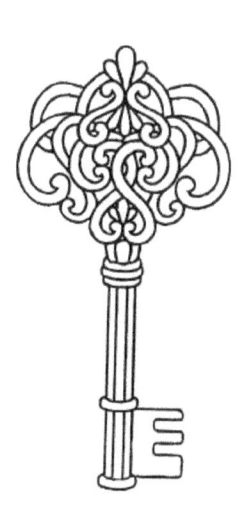

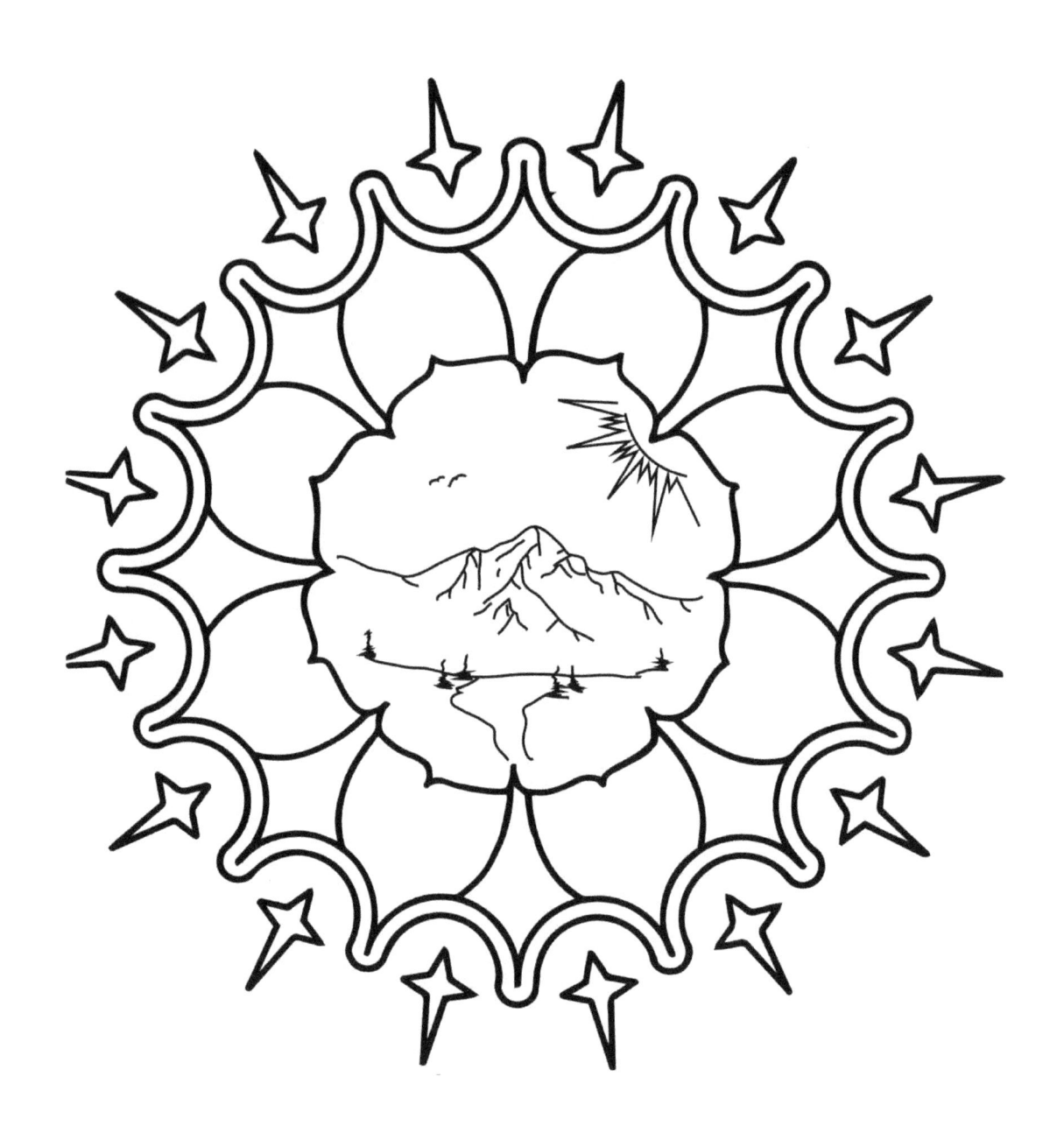

PART III: INTERMEDIATE ELEMENTARY STORIES

MOVING ON

It was time to say goodbye.

Bantu was leaving the village and school that had been home for so many years. No longer would he see the people who had lived and worked beside him for so long. There was nothing left for him in this place any more. He had reached the end of what he would be able to do here. He had to move on.

Bantu had so many feelings about leaving. Sometimes those feeling were like a roller coaster, bringing him up and then crashing down quickly without stopping. Sometimes those feelings flooded him like a rain storm, all at the same time. At one moment he felt sad about leaving all that he had known and done for so long. At another moment, he felt excited about what lay ahead, thinking of it as a new adventure that could be filled with great things.

Then his thoughts shifted again, and he felt concerned that maybe he had failed, and had not done enough in this place, and then he became worried that perhaps he would not be able to do what would be expected of him in the new place. But time was passing and he had to go, whether he liked it or not.

What could he do, Bantu thought, to calm his fears and take that next step? He wanted to be able to fill his mind with positive thoughts, look ahead instead of behind, and remember the good. Bantu sighed. It was harder to calm his fears and quiet his mind than he thought it would be.

"I guess, I will just have to keep on trying," Bantu said to himself. He tried taking a long walk. His mind kept shifting back to his worries and fears.

"This isn't working," he said. Then he decided to focus on the trees he saw while walking. When he did that, he started to notice the colors in the trees, the way the wind moved the branches and leaves, and the birds that flew to the branches and sang while he passed them. While he was noticing all this, he did not have any thoughts about his troubles. His breath felt lighter, and his steps felt strong.

"Wow, I feel better," he said. "By looking at what is around me, I gave my mind a rest!"

After his walk, he felt better for a while, but then his roller coaster feelings came back again.

"What else can I do to help me feel better?" he thought. He began to hum a tune, and then he started to sing the words. He filled his lungs with air and started to sing louder, holding notes longer. His body began to move with his own music and he felt happy and free.

"I feel great," Bantu said.

Bantu remained happy for a while, and then, the bad feelings started to return. He began to feel discouraged.

"I will never get free of these bad feelings," he said.

Bantu sat quietly, and thought about what had helped him before. He realized that he had to let his mind pay attention to what he is doing in this moment rather than worry about what lies ahead or what he might not have done in the past.

He closed his eyes and started to breathe.

He stretched his body and opened his heart to the sky.

He twisted his body to get rid of his sadness and fear.

He moved his body up and down, side to side, lowering his head, and then lifting it again.

When he felt finished, he lay down and relaxed.

His body felt good and his mind felt rested.

He knew that he would be ok, whatever happened.

He had made changes before and had done things that were hard for him, and it all worked out. It will work out again this time too.

PART III: INTERMEDIATE ELEMENTARY STORIES

DISCUSSION QUESTIONS FOR "MOVING ON"

1. Have you ever had to make a change like Bantu?
2. We can experience many feelings about a situation at one time. What are the feelings that Bantu experienced? (Sadness, excitement, worried.) Can you describe a situation in which you had multiple feelings at the same time?
3. What did Bantu have to do to feel better about his situation? (He had to focus his mind on the moment rather than worrying about what might happen or what happened in the past.)
4. What feeling did Bantu have at the end of the story? (He felt positive and relaxed. He felt that he would be OK, whatever happened.)

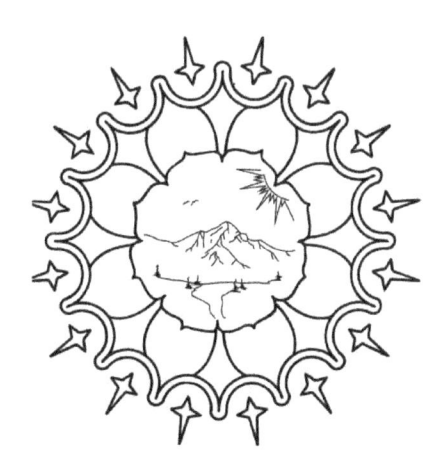

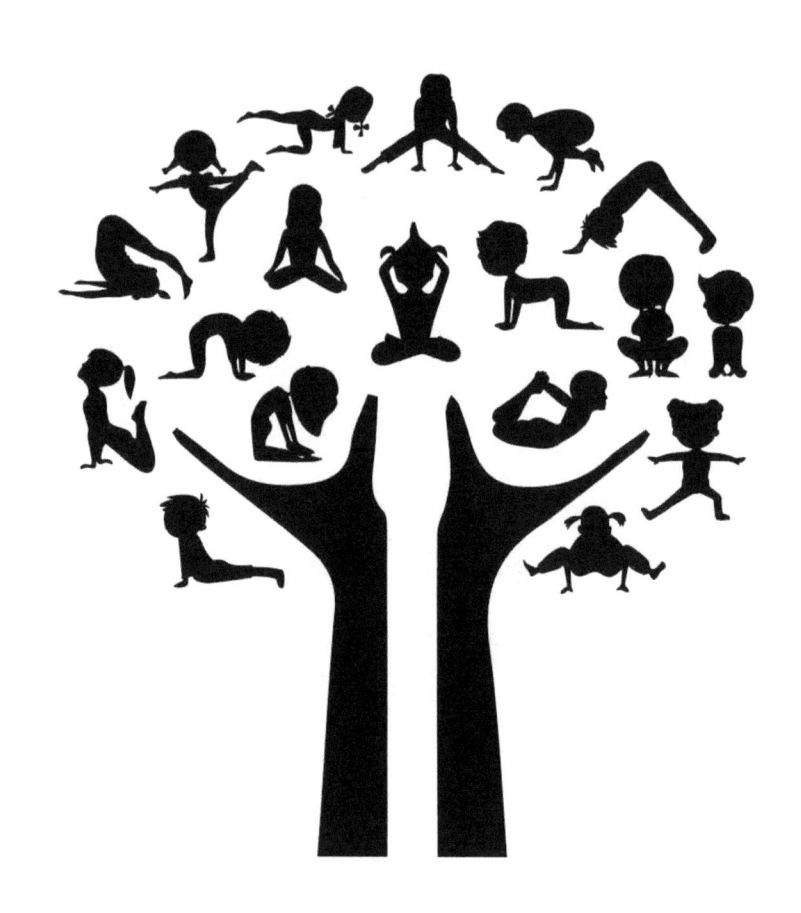

AFTERWORD

I sincerely hope that these stories will be an effective vehicle for growth for the children with whom you work. The connection of mind, body, feelings, and spirit shown in these stories have the power to lead to self-understanding, build resilience, and adopt coping skills that are vital to navigating the world as we move through life.

I am grateful to be able to share these stories with you. They represent the feelings, struggles, and conflicts of children I have had the opportunity to help, and they show strategies for healing that we explored together.

It is my hope also that you are able to use these stories to help the children in your life.

Truly Yours,
Sharon Mond

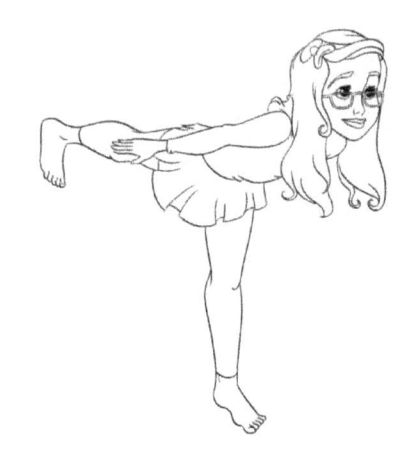

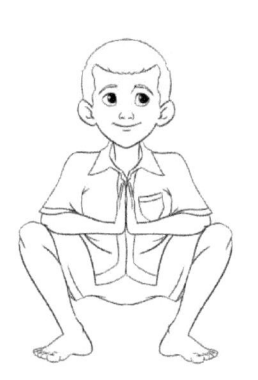

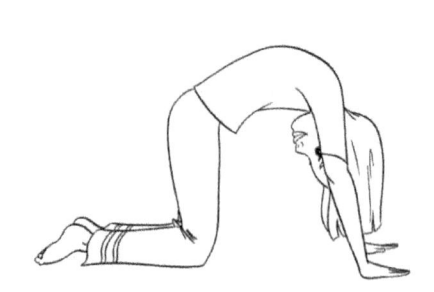

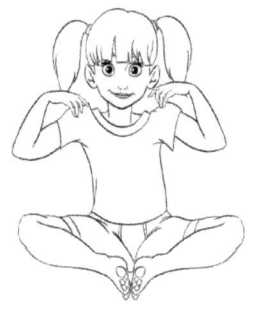

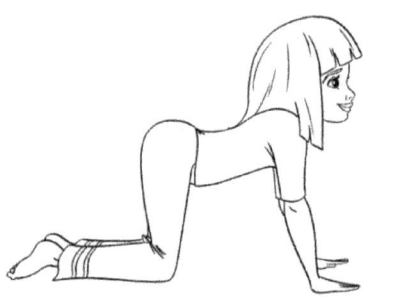

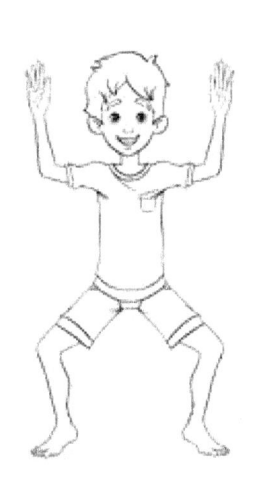

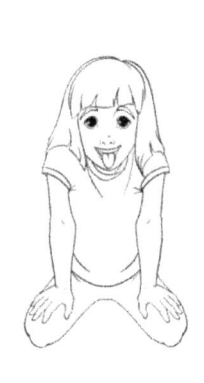

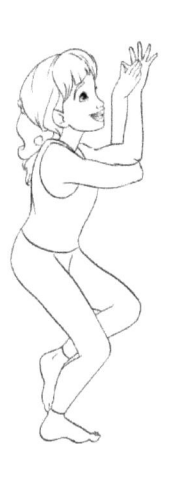

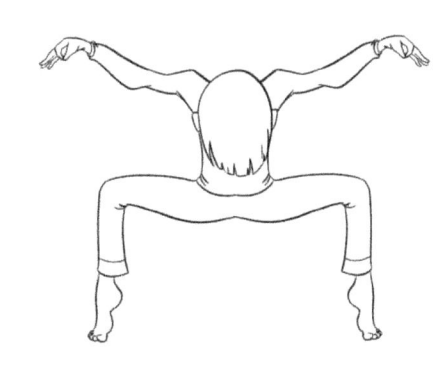

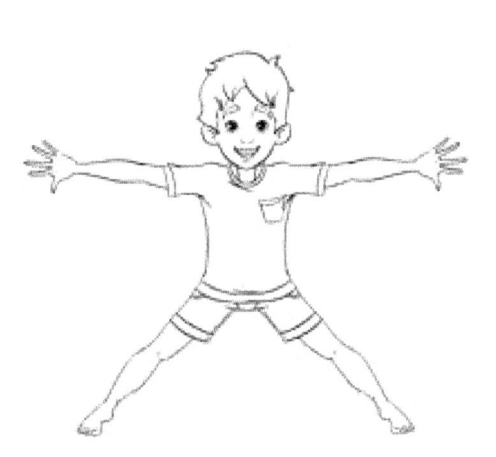

Printed in the USA
CPSIA information can be obtained
at www.ICGtesting.com
LVHW071109221223
767112LV00085B/3486